Last Minute Intercollegiat MRCS Clinical Problem Solving EMQs

Editor

MARC GLADMAN

Contributors

Toby Hammond
Ben Ollivere
Greg Shaw
Subash Vasudevan

PasTest

Dedicated to your BRITISH MEDICAL ASSOCIATION

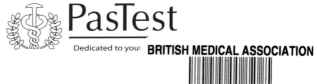

© 2006 PASTEST LTD
Egerton Court
Parkgate Estate
Knutsford
Cheshire
WA16 8DX

Telephone: 01565 752000

First Published 2006

ISBN: 1 905635 07 9
ISBN: 978 1905635 078

A catalogue record for this book is available from the British Library.

The information contained within this book was obtained by the author from reliable sources. However, while every effort has been made to ensure its accuracy, no responsibility for loss, damage or injury occasioned to any person acting or refraining from action as a result of information contained herein can be accepted by the publishers or authors.

PasTest Revision Books and Intensive Courses

PasTest has been established in the field of postgraduate medical education since 1972, providing revision books and intensive study courses for doctors preparing for their professional examinations.

Books and courses are available for the following specialties:

MRCGP, MRCP Parts 1 and 2, MRCPCH Parts 1 and 2, MRCPsych, MRCS, MRCOG Parts 1 and 2, DRCOG, DCH, FRCA, PLAB Parts 1 and 2.

For further details contact:

PasTest, Freepost, Knutsford, Cheshire WA16 7BR

Tel: 01565 752000   **Fax: 01565 650264**
www.pastest.co.uk   **enquiries@pastest.co.uk**

Text prepared by Type Study, Scarborough, North Yorkshire

Printed and bound in the UK by Cambridge University Press, Cambridge

CONTENTS

PREFACE

This book is intended for use by candidates preparing for the clinical problem solving paper (Part 2) of the Intercollegiate MRCS examination. This is a 3-hour examination consisting of 180 'extended matching items'. The questions consist of a theme, a list of options (in alphabetical order), an instruction and a variable number of clinical situations. For each of these clinical situations, the single most likely option should be selected by the candidate from the list of options.

The questions in this text have been specifically designed to cover *all* aspects of the latest Intercollegiate MRCS syllabus (January 2006). The syllabus is divided into three sections: (i) applied basic sciences; (ii) principles of surgery-in-general; and (iii) surgical specialties. Currently, the latter two areas are examined in the clinical problem solving paper (Part 2) of the Intercollegiate MRCS. Accordingly, this book is divided into the same sections so that revision and examination practice can be focused around specific topics as required.

In addition to a sound knowledge base in those topics listed in the syllabus, repeated practise of large numbers of extended matching questions (EMQs) is considered the most useful preparation for the examination by successful candidates. Accordingly, this book forms part of a trilogy of books published by PasTest aimed at steering prospective candidates through this section of the examination. It is suggested, therefore, that this book be used in conjunction with the other books in this series (*Intercollegiate MRCS Clinical Problem Solving EMQs* Volumes 1 and 2 and *Intercollegiate MRCS EMQ Practice Papers*).

This book may be used at any stage while studying for Part 2 of the Intercollegiate MRCS examination, although it is hoped that it will prove particularly useful for 'last minute' preparation. As such, the aims of the book are two-fold. Firstly, to provide a selection of EMQs representative of those that will be encountered in the paper which the candidate can attempt during the final preparations for the examination. Just as in the Part 2 examination itself, the level of difficulty of individual items is variable. Accordingly, the items in this book vary in their level of difficulty. For identification purposes, the more difficult items are disclosed to the candidate in the answer section. Such items have been assigned a double asterix (**). Secondly, the book aims to emphasise 'key points' for each of the themes covered. These are provided in preference to a detailed explanation of individual answers and have been specifically constructed to focus attention on aspects considered to be of particular importance. In addition, reference to the relevant section of *Essential Revision Notes for Intercollegiate MRCS* Books 1 and 2 published by PasTest is provided so that candidates may consult a more definitive text to supplement their knowledge if required.

Marc A Gladman
Editor

CONTRIBUTORS

EDITOR

Marc A Gladman PhD, MRCOG, MRCS (Eng)

Specialist Registrar in General Surgery
Centre for Academic Surgery
Institute of Cell and Molecular Science
Bart's and The London
Queen Mary's School of Medicine and Dentistry
University of London
London

CONTRIBUTORS

Toby Hammond MB ChB, MRCS (Eng)

Specialist Registrar in General Surgery
Homerton University Hospital NHS Trust
London

Ben Ollivere MA (Oxon), MB BS, MRCS

Specialist Registrar in Trauma and Orthopaedic Surgery
Norfolk and Norwich University Hospital NHS Trust
Norwich

Greg Shaw BSc (Hons), MRCS (Eng)

Specialist Registrar in Urology
North Thames Rotation

Subash P Vasudevan MRCS

Clinical Research and Teaching Fellow
Centre for Academic Surgery
Royal London Hospital
London

EXAMINATION TECHNIQUE

The written section of the new Intercollegiate Membership examination of the Surgical Royal Colleges of Great Britain and Ireland has undergone recent revision (2004) and now comprises two written papers: Part 1 for Applied Basic Sciences (ABS) and Part 2 for Clinical Problem Solving (CPS). The Part 1 ABS paper consists of multiple true/false questions only. Candidates are allowed 3 hours for the paper. The Part 2 CPS consists of extended matching questions only and is presently 2½ hours in length but from April 2005 will last 3 hours.

Pacing yourself accurately during the examination to finish on time, or with time to spare, is essential. There are two common mistakes that cause good candidates to fail the MRCS written examinations. These are neglecting to read the directions and questions carefully enough and failing to fill in the computer answer card properly. You must read the instructions given to candidates at the beginning of each section of the paper to ensure that you complete the answer sheet correctly.

You must also decide on a strategy to follow with regard to marking your answer sheet. The answer sheet is read by an automatic document reader and transfers the information to a computer. It is critical that the answer sheet is filled in clearly and accurately using the pencils provided. Failure to fill in your name and your examination correctly could result in the rejection of your paper.

Some candidates mark their answers directly onto the computer sheet as they go through the questions, others prefer to make a note of their answers on the question paper, and reserve time at the end to transfer their answers onto the computer sheet. If you choose the first method, there is a chance that you may decide to change your answer after a second reading. If you do change your answer on the computer sheet, you must ensure that your original is thoroughly erased. If you choose the second method, make sure that you allow enough time to transfer your answers methodically onto the computer sheet, as rushing at this stage could introduce some costly mistakes. You will find it less confusing if you transfer your marks after you have completed each section of the examination. You must ensure that you have left sufficient time to transfer your marks from the question paper to the answer sheet. You should also be aware that no additional time will be given at the end of the examination to allow you to transfer your marks.

If you find that you have time left at the end of the examination, there can be a temptation to re-read your answers time and time again, so that even those that seemed straightforward will start to look less convincing. In this situation, first thoughts are usually best, don't alter your initial answers unless you are sure.

You must also ensure that you read the question (both stem and items) carefully. Regard each item as being independent of every other item, each referring to a specific quantum of knowledge. For the CPS section, it is important to choose the *most likely* answer as there may be more than one 'correct' answer. For every correct answer you will gain a mark (+1). Marks will not be deducted for a wrong answer. Equally, you will not gain a mark if you mark both true and false.

For this reason you should answer evey question as you have nothing to lose. If you do not know the answer to a question, you should make an educated guess – you may well get the answer right and gain a mark.

If you feel that you need to spend more time puzzling over a question, leave it and, if you have time, return to it. Make sure you have collected all the marks you can before you come back to any difficult questions.
Multiple choice questions are not designed to trick you or confuse you, they are designed to test your knowledge of medicine. Accept each question at face value.

The aim of this book is to give you practice and therefore aid revision for the Part 2 CPS paper. The broad range of questions is to test your knowledge on specific subjects.

Working through the questions in this book will help you to identify your weak subject areas. In the last few weeks before the exam it will be important for you to avoid minor unimportant areas and concentrate on the most important subject areas covered in the exam.

ABBREVIATIONS

AAA	abdominal aortic aneurysm
ABPI	ankle-brachial pressure index
ACE	antegrade continence enema
ACTH	adrenocorticotropic hormone
ADH	antidiuretic hormone
A&E	Accident and Emergency
AFP	α-fetoprotein
ALP	alkaline phosphatase
ARDS	acute respiratory distress syndrome
ASA	American Society of Anaesthesiologists
AST	Aspartate transaminase
ATLS	Advanced Trauma Life Support
BCG	bacille Calmette Guérin
BiPAP	biphasic positive airways pressure
BIPP	bismuth iodoform paraffin paste
BMI	body mass index
BP	blood pressure
bpm	beats per minute
CA19-9	cancer antigen 19-9
CA125	cancer antigen 125
CABG	carotid artery bypass graft
CBD	common bile duct
CCRiSP	Care of the critically ill surgical patient
CEA	carcinoembryonic antigen
CIPO	chronic idiopathic intestinal pseudo-obstruction
CMV	continuous mandatory ventilation
CPAP	continuous positive airways pressure
CSF	cerebrospinal fluid
CT	computed tomography
CVA	cerebrovascular accident
CVH	chronic venous hypertension
CVP	central venous pressure
DCIS	ductal carcinoma in situ
DoH	Department of Health
DPL	diagnostic peritoneal lavage
ECG	electrocardiogram
ENT	ear, nose and throat
ERCP	endoscopic retrograde cholangiopancreatography
ERN	Essential Revision Notes
ESR	erythrocyte sedimentation rate
EVAR	endovascular repair
EUA	examination under anaesthesia
FAST	focused assessment with sonography for trauma
FBC	full blood count
FFP	fresh frozen plasma
FNAC	fine-needle aspiration biopsy
GCS	Glasgow Coma Scale

GOO	gastric outlet obstruction
GORD	gastro-oesophageal reflux disease
GP	general practitioner
β-hCG	β-human chorionic gonadotrophin
HDU	high-dependency unit
HER	human epidermal growth factor receptor
ICU	intensive care unit
INR	international normalised ratio
IP	interphalangeal
IPSS	International Prostate Scoring System
IVU	intravenous urogram
JVP	jugular venous pressure
KUB	kidney ureter bladder
LDH	Lactate dehydrogenase
LFT	liver function test
LHRH	luteinising hormone-releasing hormone
LUT	lower urinary tract
MODS	multiple organ dysfunction syndrome
MRA	magnetic resonance angiography
MRCP	magnetic retrograde cholangiopancreatography
MRCS	Membership of the Royal College of Surgeons
MRI	magnetic resonance imaging
MTP	metatarsalphalangeal
NEC	necrotising enterocolitis
NHS	National Health Service
NHSBSP	National Health Service Breast Screening Programme
NICE	National Institute for Health and Clinical Excellence
NIV	non-invasive ventilatory
NMSC	non-melanoma skin cancer
NSAID	non-steroidal anti-inflammatory drug
NSF	National Service Framework
OPSS	overwhelming post-splenectomy sepsis
ORIF	open-reduction internal fixation
$p_a(CO_2)$	arterial partial pressure of carbon dioxide
$p_a(O_2)$	arterial partial pressure of oxygen
PCA	patient-controlled analgesia
PEG	percutaneous endoscopic gastrostomy
PPI	protein-pump inhibitor
PSA	prostate-specific antigen
PTH	parathyroid hormone
RCT	randomised controlled trial
ROLL	radioisotope occult lesion localisation
RPLND	retroperitoneal lymph node dissection
RUQ	right upper quadrant
$S_a(O_2)$	arterial oxygen saturation
SHO	senior house officer
SIADH	syndrome of inappropriate antidiuretic hormone secretion
SMR	submucous resection
SIRS	systemic inflammatory response

TSH	thyroid-stimulating hormone
TIA	transient ischaemic attack
TURP	transurethral resection of the prostate
U&E	urea and electrolytes
WCC	white cell count
WFSA	World Federation of Societies of Anaesthesiology
WHO	World Health Organization

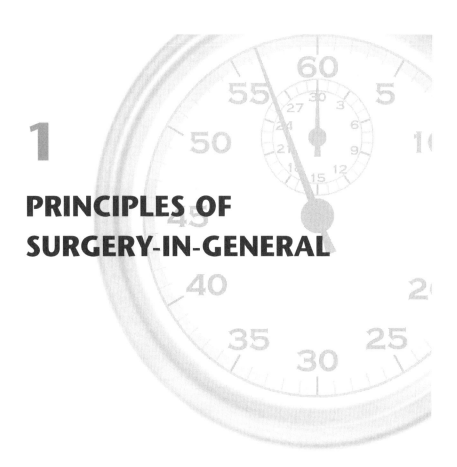

1

PRINCIPLES OF
SURGERY-IN-GENERAL

Note: Cross references in this book noting 'ERN MRCS Book 1' and 'ERN MRCS Book 2' refer to *Essential Revision Notes for Intercollegiate MRCS Books 1 and 2*. Published by PasTest. ISBN: (Book 1) 1904627366; (Book 2) 1904627374.

Note: The items in this book vary in their level of difficulty. The more difficult items are marked with a double asterix (**) in the answer section.

PERIOPERATIVE CARE

1 THEME: PREOPERATIVE FITNESS FOR SURGERY 1

A Electrocardiogram (ECG) alone
B ECG and urea and electrolytes (U&E)
C ECG, U&E, and full blood count (FBC)
D FBC, ECG, U&E and chest X-ray
E FBC, ECG, U&E, chest X-ray and lung function tests
F FBC and U&Es
G No investigation required
H Urea and electrolytes alone

From the list above pick the single most appropriate answer listing the obligatory tests required for the following clinical scenarios. The items may be used once, more than once or not at all.

☐ 1 A 4-year-old boy undergoing an elective repair of a ventriculoseptal defect, American Society of Anaesthesiologists (ASA) grade 1.

☐ 2 A 69-year-old woman booked for an elective total hip replacement with a past medical history of left ventricular failure, limiting her exercise tolerance to 180 metres (200 yards).

☐ 3 A 9-year-old boy with moderate asthma undergoing an elective tonsillectomy.

1 PREOPERATIVE FITNESS FOR SURGERY 1

1**   **D – FBC, ECG, U&E and chest X-ray**

2   **C – ECG, U&E and FBC**

3   **G – No investigations required**

- See ERN MRCS Book 1, Chapter 6, section 1 and the National Institute for Health and Clinical Excellence (NICE) guidelines *CG3 – Preoperative tests* (www.nice.org.uk/page.aspx?o=73376).

- All patients undergoing cardiovascular surgery require FBC, U&E, ECG and chest X-ray, regardless of other risk factors.

- Although commonly performed, chest X-ray is not a requirement for patients with limiting cardiovascular disease (ASA grade 3).

- Children do not require any routine investigations unless they are likely to have sickle cell disease, are undergoing neurological or cardiovascular surgery, or are known to have a life-threatening disease.

2 THEME: PREOPERATIVE FITNESS FOR SURGERY 2

A   ECG alone
B   ECG and U&E
C   ECG, U&E and full blood count
D   FBC alone
E   FBC and U&E
F   FBC, U&E, ECG and chest X-ray
G   FBC, U&E, ECG, chest X-ray and lung function tests
H   No investigation required
I   U&Es only

From the list above pick the single most appropriate answer containing the obligatory tests required for the following clinical scenarios. The items may be used once, more than once or not at all.

☐ 1   A 75-year-old man with chronic renal impairment (ASA grade 3) undergoing an elective hernia repair.

☐ 2   A 43-year-old woman undergoing elective right hemicolectomy for colorectal cancer. She is otherwise fit and well.

☐ 3   A 56-year-old man with a past history of angina undergoing elective right inguinal hernia repair (day case). He has no limitation to his exercise tolerance.

2   PREOPERATIVE FITNESS FOR SURGERY 2

1**   **B – ECG and U&E**
Hernia repair is 'intermediate surgery'. FBC is *not* considered mandatory.

2   **D – FBC alone**

3   **A – ECG alone**
ECG alone is the answer as this man is ASA grade 2 (cardiovascular) and undergoing 'intermediate surgery'.

- See ERN MRCS Book 1, Chapter 6, section 1 and the NICE guidelines *CG3 – Preoperative tests* (www.nice.org.uk/page.aspx?o=73376).

- FBC is infrequently recommended for minor and intermediate surgery, although it is often listed as a test 'to be considered'.

- Group and save has not been explicitly dealt with in the NICE guidelines.

3 THEME: PERIOPERATIVE MANAGEMENT OF ASSOCIATED CARDIORESPIRATORY DISEASE

A   Administration of of β_2-agonist at induction
B   Administration of β-blockers
C   Administration of intravenous digoxin
D   Aggressive fluid resuscitation
E   Avoidance of opioid analgesia
F   Consideration of spinal anaesthesia
G   Delay surgery for 3 months
H   Diuretic therapy
I   Endocarditis prophylaxis
J   Humidified oxygen therapy
K   Post-operative chest physiotherapy
L   Titration of intravenous fluids to central venous pressure (CVP) measurements

The following scenarios all refer to issues concerning the perioperative management of cardiorespiratory disease. Select the single most appropriate action from the list above. The items may be used once, more than once or not at all.

1   A 62-year-old man attends the preoperative assessment clinic 1 week prior to his scheduled laparoscopic cholecystectomy. The patient informs you that he was only recently discharged from the hospital following an admission for myocardial infarction.

2   A 53-year-old woman is due to undergo an emergency laparotomy for a suspected perforated duodenal ulcer. She has a body mass index (BMI) of 35, and her past medical history includes obstructive sleep apnoea.

3   A 74-year-old woman with a prosthetic aortic valve is admitted to the hospital ward 3 days prior to an elective anterior resection for rectal carcinoma, as she needs to be on intravenous heparin while her warfarin is stopped.

4   You are on call and the ward sister asks you to review a 69-year-old man with poor urine output. He has recently undergone an emergency Hartmann's procedure for a perforated sigmoid colon secondary to diverticular disease, and his past medical history includes ischaemic heart disease. Examination reveals a pulse rate of 114 beats per minute (bpm), systolic blood pressure (BP) of 100 mmHg, gross peripheral oedema and 30 ml urine output over the past 3 hours. Serum albumin is 18 g/l.

3 PERIOPERATIVE MANAGEMENT OF ASSOCIATED CARDIORESPIRATORY DISEASE

1   **G – Delay surgery for 3 months**
This is because there is a 4–6% risk of perioperative reinfarction.

2**   **E – Avoidance of opioid analgesia**

3   **I – Endocarditis prophylaxis**
Indicated in patients with prosthetic heart valves, previous endocarditis, mitral valve regurgitation and hypertrophic obstructive cardiomyopathy.

4**   **L – Titration of intravenous fluids to CVP measurements**

Perioperative management of cardiovascular disease:

- See ERN MRCS Book 1, Chapter 6, section 2.2.

- Generally, cardiac medications should not be stopped before surgery.

- Post-operative management of such patients includes adequate analgesia, supplemental oxygen therapy, maintenance of 'euvolaemia' with or without intravenous CVP monitoring.

Perioperative management of respiratory disease:

- See ERN MRCS Book 1, Chapter 6, section 2.3.

- Cessation of smoking, delaying surgery in the event of preoperative chest infection and adequate post-operative analgesia and chest physiotherapy may reduce the risk of respiratory complications post-operatively.

4   THEME: CESSATION OF MEDICATION

A	Convert from intravenous to oral route
B	Do **not** cease medication
C	Gradual withdrawal of medication
D	Immediate cessation of medication
E	Stop for 1 week preoperatively
F	Stop for 4 days preoperatively
G	Stop for 4 days preoperatively, and replace with rapidly reversible equivalent
H	Stop for 48 hours preoperatively

The following scenarios all refer to issues concerning the cessation of medication prior to surgery. Select the single most appropriate answer from the list above. The items may be used once, more than once or not at all.

1 A 62-year-old man is on warfarin, as part of the management of atrial fibrillation. He is on the waiting list for a laparoscopic cholecystectomy.

2 A 74-year-old woman is on clopidogrel, as part of the management of ischaemic heart disease. She is on the waiting list for a reversal of Hartmann's procedure.

3 A 21-year-old man attends Accident and Emergency (A&E) with abdominal pain and the passage of bloody motions up to seven times per day. As part of his management, he is started on intravenous hydrocortisone. Following 2 days of conservative management, the patient's symptoms have only marginally improved, and stool cultures are positive for *Escherichia coli* O157:H7.

4   CESSATION OF MEDICATION

1   **F – Stop for 4 days preoperatively**
Invasive surgery is generally safe (from major haemorrhagic complications) when the international normalised ratio (INR) < 1.5.

2   **E – Stop for 1 week preoperatively**
Applies to other antiplatelet drugs as well.

3**   **D – Immediate cessation of medication**
This patient has infective *not* ulcerative colitis.

- See ERN MRCS Book 1, Chapter 6, section 2.1.

- Systemic corticosteroids can be stopped abruptly in those who are unlikely to relapse and who have received treatment for < 3 weeks, otherwise gradual withdrawal should be performed.

- Metformin should be stopped 48 hours preoperatively as it can cause lactic acidosis.

5 THEME: CONSENT FOR SURGERY

A   Advance refusal
B   Battery
C   Best interests (treatment in) under common law
D   Consent for medical research
E   Implied consent (assent)
F   Informed consent
G   Negligence
H   Parental consent
I   Treatment under the Mental Health Act
J   Ward of court

The following scenarios all refer to issues concerning informed consent. Select the single most appropriate answer from the list above. The items may be used once, more than once or not at all.

1   A 20-year-old woman with severe right iliac fossa pain, but no signs of sepsis, underwent a diagnostic laparoscopy plus proceed to further surgery as required. At the time of the operation, no macroscopic organic pathology could be identified, but the surgeon proceeded to remove the appendix via the open approach in case of mucosal inflammation. The pathology report later revealed the appendix to be normal. Legal action was taken by the patient against the surgeon.

2   A 46-year-old man underwent proctoscopic injection sclerotherapy of grade II haemorrhoids in the surgical clinic. He developed acute pelvic discomfort at the time of injection, followed by urgency, dysuria, fever, and aching in the left testis. His symptoms settled with antibiotics and anti-inflammatory analgesics, but he takes legal action, claiming he was not informed of the risks of the procedure.

3   An 18-year-old man is brought into A&E following an assault. He is unconscious and severely haemodynamically unstable with a stab wound to the right hypochondrium. Following intubation and ventilation, the patient is immediately taken to the operating room for an emergency laparotomy.

5   CONSENT FOR SURGERY

1   B – Battery
This is violation of civil law that forbids intentionally touching another person without their consent. In this situation, harm can be construed as the moral violation of the patient's right to exercise autonomous control over procedures performed on their body.

2**   G – Negligence
This is failure of the professional duty of the surgeon to adequately inform patients about a chosen procedure's complications and any appropriate alternatives. In this scenario, the patient could argue that he would not of consented to the procedure had he known the risks.

3   C – Best interests (treatment in) under common law

- See ERN MRCS Book 1, Chapter 6, section 2.1; Department of Health, policy and guidance, *Health and social care topics* (www.dh.gov.uk/PolicyAndGuidance/HealthAndSocialCareTopics); General Medical Council, *Seeking patients' consent: the ethical considerations* (www.gmc-uk.org/guidance/archivelibrary/consent.asp).

- Informed consent is the process whereby a mentally competent patient agrees to undergo a procedure after discussion of the indications, alternatives, potential side effects and complications.

6 THEME: LOCAL ANAESTHETICS – TYPES AND DOSAGES

A	3 ml	H	Benzocaine
B	7 ml	I	Bupivicaine
C	8 ml	J	Cocaine
D	11 ml	K	Lidocaine
E	16 ml	L	Lidocaine + adrenaline
F	20 ml	M	Prilocaine
G	Amethocaine	N	Prilocaine + adrenaline

The following scenarios all refer to issues concerning local anaesthesia. Select the most appropriate answer from the list above. The items may be used once, more than once or not at all.

1 A 20-year-old man weighing 80 kg attends the day-stay surgical unit for excision of a small lipoma on his right thigh. Choose the anaesthetic agent of choice.

2 While closing the layers of the abdominal wall following an appendicectomy on a 40 kg child, the consultant anaesthetist requests that you infiltrate the wound with 0.5% bupivacaine. Select the appropriate safe volume to be administered.

3 A 66-year-old woman weighing 75 kg attends the day-stay surgical unit for a wedge excision of an ingrowing toenail. The consultant surgeon asks you to perform a ring-block. Select the maximum safe volume of the most commonly used anaesthetic agent (concentration 2%).

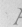

6 LOCAL ANAESTHETICS – TYPES AND DOSAGES

1   **L – Lidocaine + adrenaline**

2   **E – 16 ml**

3**   **D – 11 ml**

- See ERN MRCS Book 1, Chapter 6, section 4.1.

- Lidocaine is the most commonly used anaesthetic agent, prilocaine is the least toxic agent and safest for intravenous administration, and bupivacaine has a high affinity for cardiac muscle cells, which can lead to fatal arrhythmias. Therefore bupivacaine is contraindicated for intravenous use.

- To calculate the number of mg/ml in a dose percentage simply multiply the strength in per cent by 10 (or just move the decimal point one digit to the right), eg a 1% solution equates to 10 mg/ml of the active ingredient.

  The table below gives the commonly used anaesthetic agents, their safe dosages and duration of action.

Anaesthetic agent	Dosage ceiling	Duration of action
Lidocaine (Xylocaine)	7.0 mg/kg with adrenaline 3.0 mg/kg without adrenaline	Medium (30–90 minutes)
Bupivacaine (Marcain)	2.0 mg/kg	Long (120–240 minutes)
Prilocaine	6.0 mg/kg	Medium (30–90 minutes)
Cocaine	2.0 mg/kg	Medium (30–60 minutes)

7   THEME: MONITORING THE ANAESTHETISED PATIENT

A   Capnograph, central venous pressure, clinical observation, ECG, expired tidal volume, invasive blood pressure, pulse oximeter, pulmonary artery flotation catheter, spirometry, urometer

B   Capnograph, central venous pressure, clinical observation, ECG, expired tidal volume, invasive blood pressure, pulse oximeter, trans-oesophageal Doppler echocardiography, spirometry

C   Capnograph, central venous pressure, clinical observation, ECG, expired tidal volume, invasive blood pressure, pulse oximeter, trans-oesophageal Doppler echocardiography, urometer

D   Capnograph, clinical observation, ECG, expired tidal volume, invasive blood pressure, pulse oximeter

E   Capnograph, clinical observation, ECG, expired tidal volume, invasive blood pressure, pulse oximeter, trans-oesophageal Doppler echocardiography

F   Capnograph, clinical observation, ECG, expired tidal volume, non-invasive blood pressure, pulse oximeter

G   Central venous pressure, clinical observation, ECG, expired tidal volume, non-invasive blood pressure, pulse oximeter

H   Clinical observation, ECG, expired tidal volume, non-invasive blood pressure, pulse oximeter, spirometry

The following scenarios all refer to issues concerning the intra-operative monitoring of the anaesthetised patient. Select the single most appropriate answer from the list above. The items may be used once, more than once or not at all.

1   A 20-year-old man is due to undergo incision and drainage of a perianal abscess. The anaesthetist plans to support the patient's airway with a laryngeal mask.

2   A 74-year-old woman with history of ischaemic heart disease and a pre-operative left ventricular ejection fraction of 30% is due to undergo an emergency laparotomy for an obstructing mass in the transverse colon. The anaesthetist plans to carefully monitor her cardiovascular function to assist fluid management.

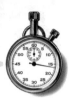

7   MONITORING THE ANAESTHETISED PATIENT

1   **D – Capnograph, clinical observation, ECG, expired tidal volume, non-invasive blood pressure, pulse oximeter**

2**   **C – Capnograph, central venous pressure, clinical observation, ECG, expired tidal volume, invasive blood pressure, pulse oximeter, transoesophageal Doppler echocardiography, urometer**

- See ERN MRCS Book 1, Chapter 6, section 4.3.

- The standards of minimal monitoring recommended by the Association of Anaesthetists of Great Britain and Ireland are:

    - The presence of an anaesthetist during the entire procedure.
    - Equipment monitoring should include an oxygen supply failure alarm, a ventilation disconnection alarm, a carbon dioxide monitor (capnograph), and a means of measuring airway pressure.
    - Patient monitoring involving (at least) capnography, clinical observation, ECG, expired tidal volume, non-invasive blood pressure, and pulse oximetry.

- Transoesophageal Doppler echocardiography is the gold standard in intraoperative monitoring of cardiovascular function in patients with cardiovascular disease (see Practice guidelines for perioperative transesophageal echocardiography. A report by the American Society of Anesthesiologists and the Society of Cardiovascular Anesthesiologists Task Force on Transesophageal Echocardiography. *Anesthesiology* 1996; 84: 986–1006).

8   THEME: POSITIONING OF PATIENT

A   Armchair
B   Lateral
C   Lateral decubitus
D   Lithotomy
E   Lloyd Davies
F   Prone
G   Prone jack-knife
H   Reverse Trendelenburg
I   Supine
J   Trendelenburg

The following scenarios all refer to operations in which specific positions are employed. Select the single most appropriate position from the list above. The items may be used once, more than once or not at all.

☐ 1   A 62-year-old man is undergoing an emergency laparotomy for an obstructing lesion in the sigmoid colon.

☐ 2   A 74-year-old woman is undergoing a right total hip replacement. ·

☐ 3   A 21-year-old man is undergoing incision and drainage of a perianal abscess.

☐ 4   A 57-year-old woman is undergoing saphenofemoral junction ligation and stripping of the long saphenous vein.

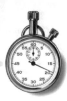

8 POSITIONING OF PATIENT

1*   **E – Lloyd Davies**
Patient is supine with hips and knees flexed to 45°. It allows excellent access to the pelvis (and simultaneously, the perineum).

2   **C – Lateral decubitus**
Patient is positioned on contralateral side to their pathology, and the table is flexed in the centre. It is employed in renal surgery (eg nephrectomy) and total hip replacements.

3   **D – Lithotomy**
Patient is supine with the hips and knees flexed to 90°.

4   **J – Trendelenburg**
Patient is supine with head-down tilt. It is usually employed for varicose vein surgery, and laparoscopic lower gastrointestinal or pelvic procedures

•   Armchair – position employed for (arthroscopic) shoulder surgery.

•   Lateral – patient is positioned on contralateral side to their pathology, eg thoracic, renal and hip surgery (although lateral decubitus is more common).

•   Prone – patient is positioned face down. It is generally employed in spinal surgery.

•   Prone jack-knife – patient in prone position with hips flexed to 90°.

•   Reverse Trendelenburg – the patient is supine, with head-up tilt, eg laparoscopic cholecystectomy and upper gastrointestinal procedures.

POST-OPERATIVE MANAGEMENT AND CRITICAL CARE

9 THEME: ARTERIAL BLOOD GASES

A   Compensated metabolic acidosis
B   Compensated metabolic alkalosis
C   Compensated respiratory acidosis
D   Compensated respiratory alkalosis
E   Metabolic acidosis and increased anion gap
F   Metabolic acidosis and normal anion gap
G   Metabolic alkalosis
H   Respiratory acidosis
I   Respiratory alkalosis

The following scenarios all refer to issues concerning arterial blood gas and serum electrolyte abnormalities. Select the single most appropriate interpretation of these blood results from the list above. The items may be used once, more than once or not at all.

☐ 1   An 82-year-old man attends A&E with severe pain in the left iliac fossa. Examination reveals tachypnoea, tachycardia and localised peritonism. His arterial blood gases are: pH 7.46, $p_a(O_2)$ 11.1 kPa, $p_a(CO_2)$ 2.6 kPa, base excess –9 mmol/l; serum blood results are: Na$^+$ 131 mmol/l, K$^+$ 3.0 mmol/l, urea 18.0 mmol/l, creatinine 198 μmol/l, Cl$^-$ 95 mmol/l, HCO$_3^-$ 13 mmol/l.

☐ 2   A 79-year-old man attends the A&E complaining of severe abdominal pain for the past 6 hours. There are no other associated symptoms or specific signs on examination. His arterial blood gases are: pH 7.33, $p_a(O_2)$ 10.4 kPa, $p_a(CO_2)$ 4.7 kPa, base excess –7.8 mmol/l; serum blood results are: Na$^+$ 136 mmol/l, K$^+$ 3.8 mmol/l, urea 12.6 mmol/l, creatinine 117 μmol/l, Cl$^-$ 96 mmol/l, HCO$_3^-$ 16 mmol/l.

☐ 3   A 57-year-old woman undergoes a laparoscopic cholecystectomy, which is converted to an open procedure; the operation takes 3 hours. Post-operatively, her arterial blood gases are: pH 7.31, $p_a(O_2)$ 8.1 kPa, $p_a(CO_2)$ 6.4 kPa, base excess –2 mmol/l; serum blood results are: Na$^+$ 140 mmol/l, K$^+$ 4.3 mmol/l, urea 7.6 mmol/l, creatinine 98 μmol/l, Cl$^-$ 100 mmol/l, HCO$_3^-$ 26 mmol/l.

9   ARTERIAL BLOOD GASES

1   **A – Compensated metabolic acidosis**

2**   **E – Metabolic acidosis and increased anion gap**

3   **H – Respiratory acidosis**

- See ERN MRCS Book 1, Chapter 7, section 2.4 and The Royal College of Surgeons, Surgical knowledge and skills website: arterial blood gases for the surgical trainee – when, how and what does it mean? (www.edu.rcsed.ac.uk/lectures/lt8.htm)

- In general pH < 7.35 indicates acidosis, and pH > 7.45 indicates alkalosis.

- The key to interpreting blood gases lies in the homoeostatic equation:

$$[H^+] + [HCO_3^-] \leftrightarrow H_2CO_3 \leftrightarrow H_2O + CO_2$$
Renal response   *Respiratory response*

- The respiratory system provides a rapid response system to maintaining normal pH levels via central pH chemoreceptors; the renal mechanism provides slower response (~48 hours) to maintaining normal pH levels by excreting H^+ ions.

- Anion gap in metabolic acidosis is calculated to differentiate between those causes that result in an increased concentration of acids (↑ anion gap) and those in which a loss of bicarbonate occurs (normal anion gap):

Anion gap = $[Na^+] + [K^+] – [Cl] – [HCO^-_3]$; normal range 8–16 mmol/l

- – *Normal anion gap*: causes include renal tubular acidosis, Addison's disease, pancreatic fistula.
- – *Increased anion gap*: causes include lactic acidosis (secondary to hypovolaemia, sepsis, ischaemia) and diabetic ketoacidosis.

10 THEME: POST-OPERATIVE HYPOTENSION

A	Cardiogenic shock
B	Class I haemorrhagic shock
C	Class II haemorrhagic shock
D	Class III haemorrhagic shock
E	Class IV haemorrhagic shock
F	Neurogenic shock
G	Non-haemorrhagic hypovolaemic shock
H	Septic shock

The following scenarios all refer to post-operative hypotension. Select the single most appropriate diagnosis from the list above. The items may be used once, more than once or not at all.

☐ 1 A 74-year-old man undergoes an anterior resection for rectal carcinoma, following a course of neoadjuvant chemoradiotherapy. On day 7 post operation he develops severe lower abdominal and rectal pain. Examination reveals a blood pressure of 80/30 mmHg, pulse rate 100 bpm and warm peripheries. He is oliguric.

☐ 2 An 81-year-old woman undergoes an emergency femoral hernia repair and small bowel resection following a 4-day history of profuse vomiting and abdominal pain. Two hours post operation she has a blood pressure of 80/60 mmHg, pulse rate 114 bpm and cold peripheries, and she is oliguric.

☐ 3 An 18-year-old man has a right femoral nail insertion following a traumatic mid-shaft femoral fracture. Post-operatively his blood pressure is 90/60 mmHg, pulse rate 125 bpm. He has cold peripheries and is oliguric.

☐ 4 A 57-year-old man undergoes an Ivor–Lewis oesophagogastrectomy for a lower-third oesophageal carcinoma. He has an epidural at the level of the fourth thoracic vertebra. Two hours post operation he has a blood pressure of 70/30 mmHg, pulse rate 60 bpm and warm peripheries, and he is oliguric.

10 POST-OPERATIVE HYPOTENSION

1 **H – Septic shock**
The primary response is a fall in systemic vascular resistance due to loss of vascular tone, vasodilatation and increased capillary permeability. Treatment involves noradrenaline infusion in parallel with fluid resuscitation.

2 **G – Non-haemorrhagic hypovolaemic shock**
Causes include acute pancreatitis, acute bowel obstruction, gastric outlet obstruction, severe gastroenteritis or prolonged thoracic or abdominal surgery.

3** **D – Class III haemorrhagic shock**

4** **F – Neurogenic shock**
In this case this is secondary to epidural analgesia. Pathophysiology includes loss of vasoconstriction and reflex tachycardia secondary to sympathetic blockade.

• See ERN MRCS Book 1, Chapter 5 (section 2.2) and Chapter 7 (sections 2.3, 3.4 and 8.1) and Chapter 8, section 2.4. See also *Advanced Trauma Life Support* (ATLS) and *Care of the Critically Ill Surgical Patient* (CCRiSP) course manuals.

11 THEME: POST-OPERATIVE RESPIRATORY FAILURE AND VENTILATORY SUPPORT

A Analgesia, chest physiotherapy and mask oxygen therapy
B Biphasic positive airways pressure
C Continuous mandatory pressure-controlled ventilation
D Continuous mandatory volume-controlled ventilation
E Continuous positive airways pressure
F Negative pressure ventilation
G Pressure support ventilation
H Synchronous intermittent mandatory ventilation

The following scenarios all refer to the diagnosis and management of respiratory compromise. Select the single most appropriate type of respiratory support from the list above. The items may be used once, more than once or not at all.

1 A 58-year-old man is being managed for severe acute pancreatitis. On day 2 post admission, the patient is severely dyspnoeic despite attempts at non-invasive ventilation. Examination reveals a respiratory rate 40 breaths/min, pulse rate 112 bpm, blood pressure 90/60 mmHg and auscultatory findings of bilateral widespread crepitations. Arterial blood gases are: pH 7.35, $p_a(O_2)$ 7.5 kPa, $p_a(CO_2)$ 7.52 kPa.

2 An 82-year-old man with a history of ischaemic heart disease undergoes an anterior resection for rectal carcinoma. On day 3 post operation he is severely dyspnoeic; examination reveals a respiratory rate 34 breaths/min, pulse rate 109 bpm, blood pressure 100/70 mmHg and auscultatory findings of bilateral mid to lower zone crepitations. Arterial blood gases on 60% inspired oxygen are: pH 7.38, $p_a(O_2)$ 8.1 kPa, $p_a(CO_2)$ 4.9 kPa.

3 A 61-year-old woman undergoes an elective laparoscopic cholecystectomy that has to be converted to an open procedure. Six hours post operation she is dyspnoeic; examination reveals a respiratory rate 28 breaths/min, pulse rate 100 bpm, blood pressure 130/70 mmHg and auscultatory findings of reduced air entry at the right base. Arterial blood gases are: pH 7.35, $p_a(O_2)$ 8.9 kPa, $p_a(CO_2)$ 4.5 kPa.

11   POST-OPERATIVE RESPIRATORY FAILURE AND VENTILATORY SUPPORT

1**   C – Continuous mandatory pressure-controlled ventilation

2   E – Continuous positive airways pressure

3   A – Analgesia, chest physiotherapy and mask oxygen therapy

- See ERN MRCS Book 1, Chapter 7, sections 4.4 and 4.5.

- Respiratory failure defined as $p_a(O_2) < 8.0$ kPa:

  - Type I: $p_a(CO_2) < 6.7$ kPa due to ventilation-perfusion mismatch → inadequate oxygenation.
  - Type II: $p_a(CO_2) > 6.7$ kPa due to inadequate ventilation (eg ↓ respiratory drive; neuromuscular pathology; thoracic wall pathology; airway/lung pathology.

- Step-wise management:

1   Humidified oxygen therapy (aim for $SaO_2 > 92\%$), adequate analgesia, chest physiotherapy and regular saline nebulisers.

2   Non-invasive ventilatory (NIV) support:

  - continuous positive airways pressure (CPAP)
  - biphasic positive airways pressure (BiPAP).

3   Invasive ventilatory support – indicated when NIV has failed or is unsuitable:

  - Continuous mandatory ventilation (CMV) – requires complete anaesthesia, and includes volume- or pressure-controlled ventilation.
  - Synchronous intermittent mandatory ventilation and pressure-support ventilation – allow patients to make their own respiratory effort, which is effectively 'topped-up' by the ventilator.
  - Negative pressure ventilation refers to devices that reduce the extra-thoracic pressure, such as 'iron-lungs'.

12 THEME: SURGICAL ANALGESIA

A	Epidural analgesia
B	Intravenous opioids
C	Local nerve blockade
D	Oral opioids
E	Oral paracetamol
F	Oral paracetamol and opioids
G	Oral paracetamol, opioids and non-steradal anti-inflammatory drugs (NSAIDs)
H	Oral NSAIDs
I	Patient-controlled analgesia

The following scenarios all refer to the management of post-operative pain. Select the single most appropriate type of analgesia from the list above. The items may be used once, more than once or not at all.

1 A 62-year-old man is due to undergo a left inguinal hernia repair under general anaesthesia. The patient informs you that he experienced severe groin pain in the immediate post-operative period following repair of his right inguinal hernia 2 years ago, and he asks if there is anything that can be done to avoid this complication.

2 A 71-year-old woman is due to undergo an abdominoperineal excision of rectum for a locally invasive low rectal carcinoma.

3 A 58-year-old man undergoes an elective laparoscopic cholecystectomy, which has to be converted to an open procedure.

12 SURGICAL ANALGESIA

1   C – Local nerve blockade

2**   A – Epidural analgesia
A continuous infusion of a local anaesthetic/opioid mixture is the most effective method of providing pain relief for major abdominal or thoracic surgery. Complications include:

- hypotension secondary to sympathetic blockade (3–30%)
- respiratory depression (0.2–0.4%)
- neurological sequelae (~0.07%)
- epidural abscess (~1/2000).

3   I – Patient-controlled analgesia

- See ERN MRCS Book 1, Chapter 6, section 4.4.

- The World Federation of Societies of Anaesthesiology (WFSA) Analgesic Ladder has been developed for the treatment of acute pain and steps down in contrast with the step-up approach in the WHO Analgesic Ladder (which is meant for improving pain control in patients with cancer pain):

  I – Initially, pain can be severe and may require strong intravenous opioids in combination with local anaesthetic blocks and peripherally acting drugs.
  II – Restoration of the use of the oral route to deliver analgesia. Adequate analgesia can be obtained by using combinations of peripherally acting agents and weak opioids (eg codeine, tramadol).
  III – Pain is controlled with peripherally acting agents (eg aspirin, paracetamol or NSAIDs alone).

13   THEME: FLUID MANAGEMENT

A   0.18% saline/4% dextrose at 68 ml/h
B   0.18% saline/4% dextrose at 125 ml/h
C   0.9% saline at 125 ml/h
D   125 ml/h plus ml for ml replacement of nasogastric losses
E   180 ml/h of crystalloid solution plus ml for ml replacement of nasogastric losses
F   500 ml Gelofusine bolus followed by 125 ml/h Hartmann's solution
G   1000 ml crystalloid fluid bolus followed by 125 ml/h 0.9% saline
H   Flush urethral catheter
I   Intravenous furosemide

The following scenarios all refer to patients requiring fluid support. Select the single most appropriate option from the list above. The items may be used once, more than once or not at all.

☐ 1   An 8-year-old child, weighing 25 kg, develops an ileus following an appendicectomy for a perforated appendix. The ward nurse requests for more intravenous fluids to be prescribed.

☐ 2   A 62-year-old man, weighing 70 kg, is day 2 postemergency Hartmann's operation for an obstructing sigmoid tumour. Examination of his 24-hour fluid chart reveals: 3000 ml of iv dextrose/saline, 125 ml via patient-controlled analgesia (PCA) 600 ml of antibiotic solution and 250 ml water orally, nasogastric output 4500 ml, pelvic drain 700 ml, and urine output 850 ml. His stoma has not worked and his abdomen is grossly distended. Which is the most appropriate fluid regimen?

14   THEME: ENTERAL AND PARENTERAL NUTRITION

A   Eating and drinking
B   Elemental diet
C   Feeding jejunostomy
D   Low volume, low electrolyte feed
E   Modular diet
F   Nasogastric feeding
G   Nasojejunal feeding
H   Percutaneous endoscopic gastrostomy feeding
I   Polymeric diet
J   Total parenteral nutrition

The following scenarios all refer to patients requiring nutritional support. Select the single most appropriate option from the list above. The items may be used once, more than once or not at all.

☐ 1   A 62-year-old man has been on the intensive care unit for 8 days following a severe closed head injury.

☐ 2   A 71-year-old woman with a high output proximal enterocutaneous fistula.

☐ 3   A 32-year-old man is admitted with severe exacerbation of Crohn's disease. He is being managed on maximal medical therapy for 72 hours prior to consideration for a total colectomy.

13 FLUID MANAGEMENT

1   **A** – 0.18% saline/4% dextrose at 68 ml/h

2**   **E** – 180 ml/h of crystalloid solution plus ml for ml replacement of nasogastric losses

- See ERN MRCS Book 1, Chapter 7, section 2.3.

- Normal electrolyte requirements:

    - potassium 1 mmol/kg per 24 hours (**do not** give > 40 mmol/h)
    - sodium 1.5 mmol/kg per 24 hours.

- Normal fluid requirements:

    - normal daily fluid requirements[†] + pre-existing losses + ml for ml replacement of current gastrointestinal losses (eg nasogastric/fistula/stoma output, diarrhoea)
    - [†]adults ~ 30–40 ml/kg per 24 hours
    - [†]children ~ 4 ml/kg per hour for first 10 kg body weight, plus 2 ml/kg per hour for second 10 kg body weight, plus 1 ml/kg per hour for each subsequent 1 kg body weight).

- Aim for urine output > 0.5 ml/kg per hour.

14 ENTERAL AND PARENTERAL NUTRITION

1   **G** – Nasojejunal feeding

2**   **J** – Total parenteral nutrition

3   **J** – Total parenteral nutrition

- See ERN MRCS Book 1, Chapter 6, section 2.9.

- Normal daily energy requirements are ~ 25–35 kcal/kg; in critically ill patients lipids should provide up to 50% of calories.

- Enteral feeding (oral with supplements; nasogastric/nasojejunal feeding; tube enterostomy) is preferable to parenteral feeding. It is cheaper, safer and physiological.

- Complications of enteral feeding can be 'tube related' (local pressure symptoms, enterocutaneous fistula, tube displacement or blockage) or 'feed related' (aspiration → pneumonia, diarrhoea).

- Complications of parenteral feeding can be 'catheter related' (incorrect siting of catheter, thrombophlebitis, thromboembolism, line sepsis or blockage) or 'feed related' (hyper/hypo: -glycaemia, -kalaemia, -natraemia, hypertriglyceridaemia → fatty liver, hypophosphataemia, hypercalcaemia).

15 THEME: POST-OPERATIVE CARDIORESPIRATORY COMPLICATIONS

A	Atrial fibrillation
B	Bacterial endocarditis
C	Basal atelectasis
D	Cardiogenic pulmonary oedema
E	Cardiogenic shock
F	Myocardial infarction
G	Opioid overdose
H	Pleural effusion
I	Pneumonia
J	Pulmonary embolism
K	Supraventricular tachycardia
L	Upper airway obstruction

The following scenarios all refer to patients experiencing post-operative cardiorespiratory complications. Select the single most appropriate diagnosis from the list above. The items may be used once, more than once or not at all.

1   An 82-year-old woman underwent a right hip hemiarthroplasty. On day 10 post operation she is due to go home when she suddenly collapses on the ward with severe chest pain. Examination reveals a temperature 37.2 °C, respiratory rate 40 breaths/min, pulse rate 112 bpm, blood pressure 80/40 mmHg and reduced left-sided air entry on auscultation. An electro cardiogram (ECG) reveals sinus tachycardia, and arterial blood gas results are: pH 7.34, $p_a(O_2)$ 7.4 kPa, $p_a(CO_2)$ 3.9 kPa.

2   An 18-year-old man, with a chronic history of intravenous drug misuse, underwent incision and drainage of a left groin abscess. On day 2 post operation he experiences rigors and dyspnoea. Examination reveals a temperature of 39 °C, respiratory rate 28 breaths/min, pulse rate 130 bpm, blood pressure 110/ 70 mmHg, and a diastolic murmur on cardiac auscultation.

3   A 76-year-old man undergoes an emergency laparotomy for small bowel obstruction, requiring a limited resection and primary anastomosis. He had an epidural for pain relief but this was stopped due to reactive hypotension. On day 1 post operation he is dyspnoeic; examination reveals a tempera-ture 37.4 °C, respiratory rate 30 breaths/min, pulse rate 112 bpm, blood pressure 120/80 mmHg and reduced air entry at the right lung base on auscultation. Arterial blood gas results are: pH 7.37, $p_a(O_2)$ 9.4 kPa, $p_a(CO_2)$ 5.2 kPa.

15   POST-OPERATIVE CARDIORESPIRATORY COMPLICATIONS

1   J – Pulmonary embolism

2   B – Bacterial endocarditis

3   C – Basal atelectasis

- See ERN MRCS Book 1, Chapter 6, sections 2.2 and 2.3.

- See also answer to Question 3 (on Perioperative management of associated cardiorespiratory disease).

16 THEME: POST-OPERATIVE OLIGURIA

A   Acute tubular necrosis
B   Cardiogenic shock
C   Constipation
D   Haemorrhage
E   Hepatorenal syndrome
F   Increased antidiuretic hormone (ADH) secretion
G   Myoglobinuria
H   Non-haemorrhagic hypovolaemia
I   Renal artery occlusion
J   Renal vasoconstriction
K   Sepsis
L   Third space loss
M   Tubulointerstitial nephritis
N   Urinary retention

The following scenarios all refer to patients experiencing post-operative oliguria. Select the most appropriate diagnosis from the list above. The items may be used once, more than once or not at all.

1   An 82-year-old woman underwent a pancreaticoduodenectomy for pancreatic cancer. On day 3 post operation the high-dependency unit (HDU) nurse requests more intravenous fluids, as the patient's urine output has been less than 20 ml/h for the past 3 hours. Examination reveals the patient to be grossly oedematous. Her pulse rate is 107 bpm, blood pressure 110/60 mmHg and CVP is 9 cmH$_2$O. Her serum albumin is 12 g/l.

2   A 64-year-old man is admitted with an acutely ischaemic right leg. An angiogram reveals occlusion of the right superficial femoral artery with good distal run off. Since undergoing the angiogram the urine output has been less than 10 ml/h for 3 hours. On admission his serum urea and creatinine were 12 mmol/l and 200 μmol/l, respectively.

3   A 43-year-old woman is admitted to the hospital with severe right upper quadrant (RUQ) pain, rigors and jaundice. An abdominal ultrasound reveals a calculus impacted in the common bile duct (CBD). The patient proceeds to undergo an endoscopic retrograde cholangiopancreatography (ERCP), at which the stone is removed and a sphincterotomy performed. Six hours after ERCP, the patient has a temperature of 38.5 °C, pulse rate 115 bpm, warm peripheries and a urine output of 5–10 ml for the past 2 hours.

16   POST-OPERATIVE OLIGURIA

1   **L – Third space loss**

2**   **J – Renal vasoconstriction**
NSAIDs and contrast agents → renal vasoconstriction and possible tubulointerstitial nephritis.

3   **K – Sepsis**

- See ERN MRCS Book 1, Chapter 7, section 5.

- Oliguria (100–400 ml/24 h) is common post-operatively, and is the first indicator for the development of acute renal failure.

- Acute renal failure may be:

    - pre-renal – haemorrhage, non-haemorrhagic hypovolaemia, sepsis
    - renal – acute tubular necrosis secondary to hypotension, myoglobinuria, contrast media/nephrotoxic drugs
    - post-renal – obstruction of renal tract, eg secondary urethral catheter blockage, calculus etc.

- Management of acute renal failure includes:

    - treatment of hyperkalaemia
    - identification and treatment of underlying cause (relieve urinary tract obstruction and cessation/avoidance of nephrotoxic drugs
    - strict fluid and electrolyte balance
    - early consideration of renal replacement therapy, usually haemofiltration. Neither dopamine or furosemide reduce the need for renal replacement therapy or improve mortality.

17 THEME: MISCELLANEOUS POST-OPERATIVE COMPLICATIONS

A	Compartment syndrome	I	Pneumonia
B	Deep vein thrombosis	J	Seroma formation
C	Incisional hernia	K	Small bowel obstruction
D	Lymphoedema	L	Urinary retention
E	Mesenteric ischaemia	M	Urinary tract infection
F	Occult bleeding	N	Wound dehiscence
G	Paralytic ileus	O	Wound infection
H	Pelvic abscess		

The following scenarios all refer to post-operative complications. Select the single most appropriate diagnosis from the list above. The items may be used once, more than once or not at all.

1 A 42-year-old woman presents at the surgical clinic with swelling over a recent groin wound. She was discharged from hospital 2 weeks previously following a saphenofemoral junction ligation and long saphenous stripping for varicose veins. Examination reveals a fluctuant non-tender non-erythematous swelling within the scar. There is no cough impulse.

2 An 80-year-old man underwent an elective abdominal aortic aneurysm repair 8 days ago. The ward sister asks you to review him as he has not opened his bowels since the operation and his abdomen is grossly distended. Examination reveals a non-tender but tympanic abdomen with absent bowel sounds.

3 A 64-year-old woman underwent a left total hip replacement 5 days ago. She is now complaining of severe pain and swelling along her left thigh. Examination reveals she is pyrexial with tenderness and pitting oedema along the medial aspect of the affected thigh.

18 THEME: SYSTEMIC INFLAMMATORY RESPONSE (SIRS)/MULTIPLE ORGAN DYSFUNCTION SYNDROMES (MODS)

A	Acute respiratory distress syndrome (ARDS) phase I	D	ARDS phase IV
B	ARDS phase II	E	Ebb phase
C	ARDS phase III	F	Flow phase
		G	Necrobiosis

The following questions all refer to recognised stages in the pathway of SIRS and MODS. Select the most appropriate term from the list above. The items may be used once, more than once or not at all.

1 A stage of disease progression in which the patient is in severe respiratory distress, and the chest X-ray reveals bilateral diffuse pulmonary infiltration.

2 A stage characterised by mobilisation of energy reserves and changes in cardiovascular reflex activity.

17 MISCELLANEOUS POST-OPERATIVE COMPLICATIONS

1   **J – Seroma formation**
     This is common at sites where lymphatic drainage may be disrupted
     (eg groin/axilla).

2   **G – Paralytic ileus**
     The diagnosis is differentiated from mechanical obstruction, which may
     complicate abdominal surgery (eg adhesions, suturing bowel into the
     laparotomy wound), by the absence of bowel sounds.

3** **B – Deep vein thrombosis**
     This must be excluded in any patient developing pain, swelling or
     erythema in the lower limb post-operatively. Doppler assessment of the
     deep veins is the investigation of choice.

•   See ERN MRCS Book 1, Chapter 6, sections 5.3–5.7.

18 SYSTEMIC INFLAMMATORY RESPONSE (SIRS)/MULTIPLE ORGAN DYSFUNCTION SYNDROMES (MODS)

1** **C – ARDS phase III**

2   **E – Ebb phase**

•   See ERN MRCS Book 1, Chapter 7, sections 8.2 and 8.3.

•   MODS (mortality ~60%) is the final step of the SIRS.

•   Definition of SIRS is ≥ 2 of the following:

     –   temp < 36 °C or > 38 °C
     –   pulse rate > 90 bpm
     –   respiratory rate > 20 breaths/min
     –   white cell count < 4×10^9/l or > 12×10^9/l.

•   The response to injury/physiological insult is divided into three
     responses: (i) immediate sympathetic nervous system response;
     (ii) hormonal response (pituitary gland, adrenal gland, kidney, pancreas,
     liver); and (iii) metabolic response.

•   These responses can be divided into an acute (ebb) phase (12–24
     hours), after which, if initial treatment has been successful, is the
     delayed (flow) phase (> 24 hours; peaks at 7–10 days), or, if treatment
     was unsuccessful in either phase, there is cell/tissue death and MODS.

•   ARDS (non-cardiogenic pulmonary oedema) represents the effect of SIRS
     within the lung, and is the result of a ventilatory-perfusion mismatch
     followed by eventual inadequate ventilation.

SURGICAL TECHNIQUE AND TECHNOLOGY

19 THEME: SURGICAL WOUNDS

A	Clean abrasion	F	Contaminated abrasion
B	Clean incision	G	Contaminated incision
C	Clean laceration	H	Contaminated laceration
D	Clean-contaminated incision	I	Dirty wound
E	Clean-contaminated laceration		

From the list above, select the single most appropriate name for the wounds described below. The items may be used once, more than once or not at all.

☐ 1 A 45-year-old woman undergoing a carpal tunnel release.

☐ 2 A 45-year-old patient with a low CD4 count and a high retroviral load due to AIDS undergoing a carpal tunnel release.

☐ 3 A 65-year-old man undergoing a laparotomy and distal gastrectomy for carcinoma of the stomach.

☐ 4 A 60-year-old man is knocked off his motorbike by a bus, sustaining a compound fracture of the tibia.

20 THEME: SCARS AND CONTRACTURES

A	Acne scar	E	Depressed scar
B	Atrophic scar	F	Hypertrophic scar
C	Boxcar scar	G	Keloid scar
D	Contracture	H	Normal scar

From the list above, select the single most accurate name for the scars described below. The items may be used once, more than once or not at all.

☐ 1 A 35-year-old African man who underwent excision of a sebaceous cyst 2 years ago presents with a heaped-up scar. On examination you find that the scar is still within the limits of the original incision.

☐ 2 A 23-year-old woman attends clinic complaining of the cosmesis of a scar from a wound she sustained when she fell from a ladder and cut herself as her hand smashed through a plate of glass. The laceration to her forearm crosses Langer's lines.

☐ 3 A young female patient presents to clinic. She burnt her forearm and elbow some time ago and finds that with time the movement of the elbow has become limited.

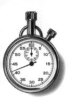

19 SURGICAL WOUNDS

1 **B – Clean incision**

2** **D – Clean-contaminated incision**
Clean procedures in an immunocompromised patient are classified as 'clean-contaminated'.

3 **D – Clean-contaminated incision**

4 **I – Dirty wound**

- See ERN MRCS Book 1, Chapter 1, section 2.1.

- Clean procedures do not require antibiotic prophylaxis.

- Clean-contaminated procedures require antibiotics at induction only.

- A procedure in which mucosa is incised but there is no spillage of contents is regarded as clean-contaminated.

- Procedures in a contaminated field require preoperative and continued post-operative doses of antibiotics.

20 SCARS AND CONTRACTURES

1 **F – Hypertrophic scar**

2** **F – Hypertrophic scar**

3 **D – Contracture**

- See ERN MRCS Book 1, Chapter 1, section 2.6.

- Contractures can be treated by excision and split-skin grafting/transposition flaps.

- Keloid scars grow outside the boundaries of the original wound.

- Incisions across Langer's lines (skin tension lines described by Carl Von Langer in 1861) should be avoided as they result in hypertrophic scars. When necessary the incisions should be oblique or S-shaped or Z-plasty should be performed.

21 THEME: SURGICAL INCISIONS

A	Evan's
B	Fergusson's
C	Flank incision
D	Gridiron
E	Kocher's
F	Lanz's
G	Mercedes
H	Pfannenstiel's

From the list above, select the name of the most appropriate incision for the scenario described below. The items may be used once, more than once or not at all.

☐ 1 A 17-year-old boy presents with an acute abdomen and a diagnosis of suspected acute appendicitis is made.

☐ 2 A 27-year-old woman undergoes an emergency Caesarean section when fetal distress develops during labour.

☐ 3 A 45-year-old man with extensive previous abdominal surgery is undergoing an open cholecystectomy. You make a simple right subcostal incision.

22 THEME: SUTURE MATERIALS

A	1/0 polyamide (Ethilon)
B	1/0 polydioxanone sulphate (PDS)
C	1/0 silk
D	3/0 polygalactin 910 (Vicryl)
E	3/0 polypropylene (Prolene)
F	4/0 catgut
G	5/0 polypropylene (Prolene)
H	6/0 polygalactin 910 (Vicryl)

From the list above, select the single most appropriate suture material for the purpose described below. The items may be used once, more than once or not at all.

☐ 1 During appendicectomy, a 30-year-old man sustains an injury to the bladder that requires closure.

☐ 2 Following adequate debridement and irrigation, a traumatic, deep scalp laceration requires surgical closure.

☐ 3 Fashioning of the distal anastomosis in a femoral–popliteal bypass.

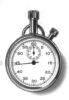

21   SURGICAL INCISIONS

1   **F – Lanz's**
This is favoured for appendicectomy, as provides superior cosmesis.

2**   **H – Pfannenstiel's**
This provides excellent access to the pelvis but *not* the upper abdominal cavity.

3   **E – Kocher's**
See ERN MRCS Book 1, Chapter 1, section 2.2.

22   SUTURE MATERIALS

1**   **D – 3/0 polygalactin 910 (Vicryl)**
Absorbable sutures are used in the urinary tract, as foreign bodies may provide a nidus for stone formation.

2   **E – 3/0 polypropylene (Prolene)**

3   **G – 5/0 polypropylene (Prolene)**

- See ERN MRCS Book 1, Chapter 1 section, 2.3.

- 1/0 or 2/0 is used for high tension.

- 3/0 is used in areas requiring good strength (eg scalp, torso, hands, etc).

- 4/0 is used in areas requiring minimal tension (eg superficial wound closure).

- 5/0 is used for areas such as the face, nose, ears, eyebrows and eyelids.

- 6/0 is used on areas requiring little tension for cosmesis.

- Polypropylene (Prolene) is the optimum choice of suture material for vascular anastomoses due to its excellent handling qualities.

- Catgut, a biological suture material, is not used any more because of the theoretical risk of transmission of prions.

23 THEME: SURGICAL INSTRUMENTS

A   Babcock's forceps
B   Ellick bulb
C   Jamshidi's needle
D   Langenbeck's retractor
E   Magill's forceps
F   Mayo scissors
G   Mosquito clamp
H   Turner–Warwick retractor

From the list above, select the most suitable instrument for the purpose described below. The items may be used once, more than once or not at all.

1   You are performing an appendicectomy under supervision and have successfully entered the peritoneal cavity in the right iliac fossa. Your registrar instructs you to deliver the caecum and appendix.

2   Your boss is allowing you to open the abdomen during a midline laparotomy for an acute abdomen. You have incised the skin and subcutaneous tissues down to the linea alba and have successfully entered the peritoneal cavity at the cicatrix. Your boss asks you to open the rest of the incision.

3   While working on surgical high-dependency unit (HDU), one of your patients requires a bone marrow biopsy to investigate a pancytopenia.

24 THEME: PRINCIPLES OF ANASTOMOSES

A   Brachiobasilic anastomosis
B   Gastrojejunal anastomosis
C   End-to-end anastomosis
D   End-to-side anastomosis
E   Enteroenteral anastomosis
F   Inlay technique
G   Parachute technique
H   Radiocephalic anastomosis
I   Side-to-side anastomosis
J   Stapled anastomosis

From the list above, select the term that is most appropriate for scenarios described below. The items may be used once, more than once or not at all.

1   A 78-year-old patient is undergoing elective repair of abdominal aortic aneurysm using a straight graft.

2   A 15-year-old patient with end-stage renal failure secondary to congenital posterior valves is awaiting transplantation and is undergoing regular haemodialysis.

3   A 45-year-old man undergoes a low anterior resection for a locally advanced adenocarcinoma with restoration of bowel continuity.

23 SURGICAL INSTRUMENTS

1 **A – Babcock's forceps**
As the area of contact at the tips is very small these forceps are useful in avoiding crush injury to the tissues

2 **F – Mayo scissors**
These are relatively heavy dissecting scissors that may be used to divide strong tissues such as the linea alba.

3** **C – Jamshidi's needle**

- The hand-held Langerbeck's retractor is good for retracting wound edges. The Turner–Warwick retractor provides an alternative and has the advantage of being a self-retaining device, consisting of a circular frame, onto which a variety of retractor blades can be attached in different positions.

- Magill's forceps are useful to position endotracheal tubes and removing foreign bodies from the upper airway.

- The Ellick bulb allows irrigation and simultaneous removal of debris/fragments (eg prostatic shavings from the bladder following transurethral resections of the prostate).

24 PRINCIPLES OF ANASTOMOSES

1 **F – Inlay technique**
This refers to the technique of positioning the graft within the native aorta to fashion the anastomosis.

2** **H – Radiocephalic anastomosis**
For haemodialysis radiocephalic arteriovenous fistulae are most commonly formed. Brachiocephalic and brachiobasilic are alternatives, but are less commonly employed.

3 **J – Stapled anastomosis**
Stapling devices have revolutionised the formation of anastomosis where access is limited.

- See ERN MRCS Book 1, Chapter 1, section 3.1.

- An anastomosis is the joining of structures (usually tubular) to maintain luminal continuity.

- Structures commonly anastomosed include: blood vessels, hollow organs (gastrointestinal and genitourinary tracts) and ducts (eg common bile duct (CBD).

- Anastomoses are at risk of rupture, leakage, infection.

25 THEME: LAPAROSCOPIC COMPLICATIONS

A Biliary peritonitis
B Capacitance coupling
C CBD injury
D Conversion to open surgery
E Injury to surrounding structures
F Intraperitoneal pressure at 20 mmHg
G Intraperitoneal pressure at 20 cmH$_2$O
H Port site herniation
I Primary haemorrhage
J Reactionary haemorrhage
K Venous gas embolism
L Visceral injury

From the list above select the single most likely complication in each of the scenarios described below. The items may be used once, more than once or not at all.

1 A 46-year-old woman develops severe abdominal pain, jaundice and tachycardia on 2 days following laparoscopic cholecystectomy.

2 A 25-year-old woman complains of painful, blistered, erythematous lesion around one of the 5-mm port site scars on day 1 post laparoscopic appendicectomy.

3 During a laparoscopic Nissen's fundoplication on an obese 40-year-old man, the anaesthetist reports difficulty maintaining the patient's blood pressure, which is now at 90/50 mmHg. There is no obvious bleeding.

25 LAPAROSCOPIC COMPLICATIONS

1 **A – Biliary peritonitis**
The development of severe abdominal pain points to this diagnosis, whereas the presence of jaundice differentiates from other causes of peritonitis post-operatively (eg viscus perforation).

2 **B – Capacitance coupling**
Defective insulation of instruments allows capacitance coupling to occur and can lead to burns at the port sites

3** **G – Intraperitoneal pressure at 20 mmHg**
High intra-abdominal pressures impair venous return and cardiac output.

- See ERN MRCS Book 1, Chapter 1, section 3.5.

- Laparoscopic surgery has many advantages over conventional surgery but is not without its complications.

- Complications may be 'general', applicable to all laparoscopic procedures or specific, applicable to individual procedures.

- The physiological consequences of a pneumoperitoneum include: decrease venous return (and thus cardiac output), increase CVP, increase peak inspiratory pressures (effect on mechanical ventilation), increase $p(CO_2)$, decrease urine output.

- Intra-abdominal pressure should *not* exceed 15 mmHg.

MANAGEMENT AND LEGAL ISSUES IN SURGERY

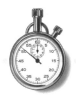

26 THEME: PRINCIPLES OF TRIAL DESIGN AND CONDUCT

A	Bias
B	Crossover design
C	Cross-sectional design
D	Double-blinding
E	Experimental study
F	Intention to treat
G	Longitudinal design
H	Null hypothesis
I	Observational study
J	Power
K	Prospective study
L	Randomisation
M	Retrospective study
N	Subgroup analysis
O	Type I error
P	Type II error

The following terms are commonly encountered with reference to clinical trial design and conduct. From the list above select the single most appropriate descriptive term for the following scenarios. The items may be used once, more than once or not at all.

☐ **1** A study that aims to investigate changes over time, with observations being taken on more than more occasion.

☐ **2** In a study investigating the analgesic effect of different medications for the treatment of post-operative pain, patients were excluded from recruitment into the study if they suffered intraoperative complications and from analysis if they developed post-operative vomiting.

☐ **3** The term used to describe a situation when the null hypothesis is rejected but no real difference is present.

26 PRINCIPLES OF TRIAL DESIGN AND CONDUCT

1   **G – Longitudinal design**

2   **A – Bias**
     These are examples of selection and exclusion bias, respectively.

3** **O – Type I error**

- See ERN MRCS Book 1, Chapter 8, section 3.1.

- Clinical trials (experiments) are designed to investigate (test) specific questions (hypotheses).

- The design may be:
  - observational (collection of information only) or experimental/interventional (events influenced and effects recorded)
  - prospective (data collected forward in time) or retrospective (data refer to past events)
  - longitudinal (investigate changes over time)
  - cross-sectional (events are observed at **one** specific point in time).

- Type I error: reject null hypothesis when no real difference is present (false positive).

- Type II error: failure to reject null hypothesis when a difference is really present (false negative).

27 THEME: TYPES OF SCIENTIFIC EVIDENCE

A   Case–control study
B   Case series
C   Cohort study
D   Controlled clinical trial
E   Cross-sectional survey
F   Non-systematic review
G   Randomised controlled trial (RCT)
H   Randomised double-blind controlled trial
I   Systematic review
J   Uncontrolled trial

From the list above select the single most appropriate term that describes the type of scientific evidence yielded in the following scenarios. The items may be used once, more than once or not at all.

1   A study describing the impact of Nissen's fundoplication on symptoms of gastro-oesophageal reflux in 150 patients.

2   A study evaluating the effect of an 'enhanced recovery programme' on post-operative recovery following abdominal surgery compared with 'standard care'. A clinical nurse specialist, who favours the 'enhanced programme' in younger patients, decides allocation into each of the two groups.

1   **B – Case series**
No intervention/control group is studied.

2**   **D – Controlled clinical trial**
Controlled to standard care but allocation is **not** randomised.

- See ERN MRCS Book 1, Chapter 8, section 3.1.

- Clinical trials should have a comparison or **control** group. Allocation to the intervention/control group should preferably be unclear to the subjects (single-blinding) and the researchers (double-blinding).

- Randomisation reduces bias due to the features of subjects that are not of interest to the study question (hypothesis), eg patient age, sex, origin, etc.

- A review of the medical literature provides a useful summary. A systematic review employs explicit methods to perform a thorough literature search and critical appraisal of individual studies and uses appropriate statistical techniques to combine the results of valid studies.

Level	Quality of evidence
1a	Systematic review of RCTs
1b	Individual RCT
2a	Systematic review of cohort studies
2b	Individual cohort study (including low-quality RCT)
3a	Systematic review of case–control studies
3b	Individual case–control study
4	Case series (and poor quality cohort and case–control studies)
5	Expert opinion without explicit critical appraisal

28 THEME: BASIC STATISTICS

A	Analysis of variance (ANOVA)
B	Chi-square test
C	Correlation
D	Kruskal–Wallis test
E	Friedman's test
F	Linear regression analysis
G	Logistic regression analysis
H	Mann–Whitney U test
I	Multiple regression analysis
J	Paired t-test
K	Power analysis
L	Regression analysis
M	Repeated measures ANOVA
N	Unpaired t-test
O	Wilcoxon's matched pairs test

The following scenarios describe various surgical studies. From the list above select the single most appropriate statistical method to analyse the study's data. The items may be used once, more than once or not at all.

1   A study evaluating two different procedures for inguinal hernia repair by comparing the proportions of patients who develop recurrence.

2   A study aiming to determine whether operative time taken for laparoscopic cholecystectomy is related to patient's body mass index, gallbladder wall thickness, common bile duct (CBD) diameter or number of calculi present in the operative specimen.

3   An interventional study comparing C-reactive protein values in 10 000 patients with Crohn's disease before and after administration of a novel 'probiotic' medication. The data **are** normally distributed.

1   **B – Chi-square test**
    Proportions, ie recurrence/non-recurrence for each procedure (2×2 table).

2** **I – Multiple regression analysis**
    Multiple continuous variables influencing operative time (dependent measure).

3   **J – Paired t-test**
    Parametric, continuous, paired data (observations – C-reactive protein level – on same individual) in two groups (before and after intervention).

- See ERN MRCS Book 1, Chapter 8, section 3.2.

- The selection of the most appropriate method of analysis requires consideration of:

    – type of data (continuous or categorical)
    – number of groups
    – independent (unpaired) or dependent (paired, ie made on the *same* individual) groups of observations.

    Appropriate tests for continuous data are shown in the table below.

	Two groups of data		More than two groups of data	
	Unpaired data	**Paired data**	**Unpaired data**	**Paired data**
Parametric (normally distributed)	t-test	Paired t-test	ANOVA	Repeated measures ANOVA
Non-parametric	Mann–Whitney U test	Wilcoxon's matched pairs test	Kruskal–Wallis test	Friedman's test

- Categorical data is analysed by comparing proportions using contingency tables (eg chi-square tests).

- Correlation and linear regression compare the *relationship* between two continuous variables.

- Multiple (dependent/outcome variable is continuous) and logistic regression (dependent/outcome variable is categorical) analysis consider more than two variables.

29 THEME: MANAGEMENT ASPECTS OF SURGICAL PRACTICE

A   Annual health check
B   Care trusts
C   Clinical audit
D   Clinical effectiveness
E   Clinical governance
F   Department of Health (DoH)
G   Foundation trusts
H   Healthcare Commission
I   Improving Outcomes guidance
J   National Institute for Health and Clinical Excellence (NICE)
K   National service frameworks (NSF)
L   National Health Service (NHS) trusts
M   Primary care trusts
N   Research
O   Strategic health authority

The following descriptions are managerial, structural and organisational terms commonly encountered within the new NHS. From the list above select the single most appropriate term. The items may be used once, more than once or not at all.

☐ 1 Ensuring that the healthcare provided is based on sound evidence.

☐ 2 Promotes improvement in the quality of the NHS and independent healthcare, and awards annual performance ratings for the NHS.

☐ 3 Introduced in 2002 to provide better integrated health and social care.

☐ 4 Responsible for providing national guidance on promoting good health and preventing and treating ill health.

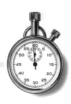

29   MANAGEMENT ASPECTS OF SURGICAL PRACTICE

1   **D – Clinical effectiveness**

2**   **H – Healthcare Commission**

3**   **B – Care trusts**

4   **J – NICE**

- See ERN MRCS Book 1, Chapter 8, section 3.1.

- Strategic health authorities manage the NHS locally and are a key link between the DoH and the NHS. Primary care trusts have taken control of local healthcare and receive budgets directly from the DoH.

- NHS trusts are independent organisations with their own managements that compete with each other. Foundation trusts have been created to devolve decision making from central government to local organisations.

- Clinical governance is the system through which NHS organisations are accountable for continuously improving the quality of their services and safeguarding high standards of care.

- The annual health check has replaced the old 'star ratings' assessment system and looks at a much broader range of issues than the targets used previously.

- Published by the NICE, Improving Outcomes guidance provides site-specific cancer guidance, which aims to support the NHS as it targets resources on the disease and co-ordinates services within and between organisations.

- NSFs are long-term strategies for improving specific areas of care. They set measurable goals within set time frames.

30   THEME: COMMUNICATION

A   Advanced refusal
B   Breaking bad news
C   Implied consent
D   Inappropriate breach of patient confidentiality
E   Informed consent
F   Legal obligation to breach patient confidentiality
G   Parental consent
H   Working in teams

The following scenarios all relate to communication between a surgeon and patient where moral, ethical and legal issues are encountered. From the list above select the single most appropriate descriptive term. The items may be used once, more than once or not at all.

1   A 61-year-old immigrant with a 3-month history of a painless neck lump attends pre-admission clinic prior to excision biopsy under general anaesthesia. On reviewing all his recent results you identify a fine-needle aspiration biopsy result of the lump, the microscopy of which reveals acid fast bacilli and the culture from which yields *Mycobacterium tuberculosis*.

2   While on a surgical ward, the receptionist asks you to speak to one of your patient's relatives, who is phoning long distance from Australia. During the course of the conversation, you inform the relative that his uncle has made an uneventful post-operative recovery but that he will need further adjuvant therapy for what turned out to be a Duke's C colorectal carcinoma.

3   You admit a 31-year-old alcoholic man with a mild head injury, which you believe was sustained innocently following a mechanical fall. The A&E sister informs you that he regularly attends the department. As you are about to leave A&E, a police constable who is present in the department tells you that the patient is often 'in trouble with the police', and he enquires whether the patient is 'drunk again' and whether his injuries are severe enough to warrant a 'head scan'.

1**   **F – Legal obligation to breach patient confidentiality**
Tuberculosis is one of 30 'notifiable diseases'.

2   **D – Inappropriate breach of patient confidentiality**
Unnecessary clinical information has been given without the patient's consent.

3   **D – Inappropriate breach of patient confidentiality**
There is no evidence that a breach of patient confidentiality is in his or the public's interest.

• See ERN MRCS Book 1, Chapter 8, section 4 and General Medical Council guidelines/section E4 of Intercollegiate MRCS examination syllabus (January 2006) for additional information.

• Breaches of patient confidentiality are **only** warranted in:

– The **public interest** where the patient poses an obvious risk to others (indeed, a legal obligation exists to report notifiable disease and suspected involvement in terrorism).
or
– The **individual's interest** when it is necessary to obtain information vital for successful treatment (eg when the physical or psychological consequences of illness prevent medical history taking) by consulting relatives.

• Generally, only those judged to be 'competent' and 16 years of age or greater can legally consent to treatment. Incompetence does not automatically follow from severe mental illness. Adolescents under 16 years may provide legal consent for surgery in exceptional circumstances, if specific criteria are met (Gillick ruling).

CLINICAL MICROBIOLOGY

31 THEME: SURGICALLY IMPORTANT MICRO-ORGANISMS

A   *Actinomyces* spp.
B   *Campylobacter jejuni*
C   *Chlamydia trachomatis*
D   *Clostridium difficile*
E   *Clostridium perfringens* (*welchii*)
F   *Clostridium tetani*
G   Coliforms
H   *Mycobacterium tuberculosis*
I   *Staphylococcus* spp.
J   *Streptococcus epidermidis*
K   *Streptococcus milleri*
L   *Streptococcus pneumoniae*
M   *Yersinia enterocolitica*

For each of the following clinical scenarios, select the most likely causative organism from the list above. The items may be used once, more than once or not at all.

▢ 1   A 6-year-old boy with a 2-day history of an upper respiratory tract infection and right iliac fossa pain undergoes appendicectomy. At operation a non-inflamed appendix was excised and numerous enlarged lymph nodes are evident in the mesoappendix.

▢ 2   A 29-year-old intravenous drug misuser presents with a 4-day history of a swollen, painful left thigh following attempted injection of the femoral vessels. On examination he has massive swelling of the left thigh with blue discoloration of the skin and obvious crepitus. Soon after admission he collapses with profound hypotension, tachycardia and fever.

▢ 3   A 76-year-old diabetic man develops obvious erythema and purulent discharge from his laparotomy wound 4 days after a Hartmann's procedure for complicated diverticulitis.

31   SURGICALLY IMPORTANT MICRO-ORGANISMS

1**   **M – *Yersinia enterocolitica***
This is the most frequent cause of mesenteric adenitis and is confirmed on serology.

2   **E – *Clostridium perfringens* (*welchii*)**
Gas gangrene is produced by the α-toxin of *C. perfringens*.

3   **G – Coliforms**

- See ERN MRCS Book 1, Chapter 2, section 3.1.

- Successful treatment of surgical infection requires knowledge of the likely offending organisms.

- 'De novo' skin infections are frequently due to skin flora (*Staph/Strep* spp.). Post-operative infections usually reflect intraoperative **contamination** of the wound.

32 THEME: APPROPRIATE ANTIMICROBIAL THERAPY

A   Benzylpenicillin
B   Cefadroxil
C   Cefalexin
D   Ceftazidime
E   Cefuroxime
F   Ciprofloxacin
G   Co-amoxiclav
H   Erythromycin
I   Flucloxacillin
J   Gentamicin
K   Metronidazole
L   No agent
M   Phenoxymethylpenicillin (penicillin V)
N   Vancomycin

For each of the following clinical scenarios, select the most appropriate anti-microbial agent for each of the following clinical scenarios. The items may be used once, more than once or not at all.

1   A 26-year-old man underwent an emergency splenectomy following a road traffic accident. Having made an uneventful recovery, you are preparing his discharge from hospital.

2   A 55-year-old man is admitted for an elective total hip replacement. He has a severe allergy to penicillin and cephalosporins. Knowing that you are preparing for the MRCS examination, your consultant asks which antibiotic should be used as prophylaxis against infection.

3   Five days following an elective left hemicolectomy, a 66-year-old woman becomes systemically septic with evidence of a paracolic abscess secondary to anastomotic leakage on a computed tomography (CT) scan. You arrange her transfer to high-dependency unit (HDU) and contact the consultant microbiologist for appropriate antimicrobial advice. In addition to metronidazole, you are instructed to commence a 'third generation' cephalosporin.

4   A 76-year-old man is undergoing induction of anaesthesia for elective abdominal aortic aneurysm repair. He has a history of severe allergy to cephalosporins. The anaesthetist asks your advice regarding administration of a suitable prophylactic antimicrobial agent.

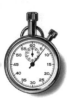

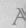

1   **M – Phenoxymethylpenicillin (penicillin V)**
Recommended for prophylaxis against pneumococci sepsis in patients with hyposplenism/asplenism.

2   **N – Vancomycin**
Single dose iv cefuroxime or iv flucloxacillin is recommended for prophylaxis or iv vancomycin if there is a history of allergy.

3   **D – Ceftazidime**

4**   **J – Gentamicin**
Single dose of iv cefuroxime *or* iv gentamicin is recommended for prophylaxis for reconstructive arterial surgery of abdomen, pelvis or legs.

•   See ERN MRCS Book 1, Chapter 2, section 6 and *British National Formulary* section 5.

•   Penicillin V/benzylpenicillin is effective against many Gram-positive aerobic organisms.

•   Flucloxacillin is effective against most staphylococci.
Ampicillin/amoxicillin is active against Gram-positive and some Gram-negative organisms but is inactivated by penicillinases including those produced by *Staphylococcus aureus* and by *Escherichia coli*.

•   'First generation' cephalosporins (cefalexin/cefadroxil) have a similar antimicrobial spectrum to the penicillins, with good Gram-positive coverage. 'Second generation' cephalosporins (cefuroxime) are less susceptible than the earlier cephalosporins to inactivation by β-lactamases. 'Third generation' cephalosporins (cefotaxime/ceftazidime) have greater activity against Gram-negative bacteria (eg pseudomonads) but at the expense of Gram-positive coverage (notably *Staphylococcus aureus*).

•   Antibiotics effective against anaerobic organisms include co-amoxiclav and metronidazole.

33 THEME: ANTIMICROBIAL RESISTANCE

A	Acquired resistance secondary to gene transfer
B	Acquired resistance secondary to mutation
C	Altered permeability
D	Cross-resistance
E	Dissociated resistance
F	Inactivation
G	Innate resistance
H	Modification of site of action

For each of the following, select the most appropriate type or mechanism of antibiotic resistance. The items may be used once, more than once or not at all.

- 1 The resistance of *Pseudomonas aeruginosa* to phenoxymethylpenicillin (penicillin V).

- 2 The resistance of staphylococci to ampicillin/amoxicillin.

34 THEME: STERILISATION AND DISINFECTION

A	121 °C for 5 minutes
B	134 °C for 3 minutes
C	Alcohol (70%)
D	Boiling water
E	Chlorhexidine
F	Ethylene oxide
G	Gamma irradiation
H	Povidone-iodine

From the list above select the single most appropriate method to achieve a safe level of decontamination for each of the following scenarios. The items may be used once, more than once or not at all.

- 1 The process to prepare surgical instruments between usage.

- 2 The preparation of clinical work surfaces.

- 3 The preparation of single-use devices constructed of plastic (eg syringes).

33 ANTIMICROBIAL RESISTANCE

1 **G – Innate resistance**
The outer membranes of pseudomonads are inherently difficult to penetrate, thus many antibiotics are ineffective (innate resistance).

2 **F – Inactivation**
This occurs due to the production of β-lactamases.

- See ERN MRCS Book 1, Chapter 2, section 6.4.

- Antibiotic resistance may be primary (innate) or secondary (acquired).

- Acquired resistance may be due to gene transfer or mutation, altered permeability (modification of proteins in outer membrane), modification of the site of action and inactivation of the antibiotic (eg β-lactamase production).

- Cross-resistance is when resistance to one antimicrobial confers resistance to others (usually chemically related).

- Dissociated resistance is when resistance to one drug is not accompanied by resistance to other similar drugs.

34 STERILISATION AND DISINFECTION

1** **B – 134 °C for 3 minutes**
Sterilisation can be achieved at 134 °C for 3 minutes or 121 °C for 15 minutes.

2 **C – Alcohol (70%)**

3 **F – Ethylene oxide**
Gamma irradiation or ethylene oxide is used in industry to sterilise medical equipment. Ethylene oxide is irritant, toxic and mutagenic. It must not be used for ventilatory equipment.

- See ERN MRCS Book 1, Chapter 2, section 5.3.

- Cleaning physically removes contamination but does not destroy microorganisms.

- Disinfection reduces the number of viable organisms but may not necessarily inactivate viruses or spores.

- Sterilisation is the complete destruction and removal of all viable microorganisms.

35 THEME: TRANSMISSION OF BLOOD-BORNE VIRUSES

A	1 in 20
B	1 in 200
C	1 in 2000
D	1 in 3
E	1 in 30
F	1 in 300
G	1 in 3000
H	1 in 6
I	1 in 60
J	1 in 600
K	1 in 6000
L	3-fold decrease
M	3-fold increase
N	6-fold decrease
O	6-fold increase
P	20-fold decrease
Q	20-fold increase

From the list above select the most appropriate rate of transmission of blood-borne viruses for the following scenarios. The items may be used once, more than once or not at all.

☐ 1 The risk of transmission of hepatitis C from an infected patient to a surgeon following a needle-stick injury.

☐ 2 The change in risk of transmission associated with 'double gloving'.

☐ 3 The risk of human immunodeficiency virus (HIV) infection following a single episode of mucocutaneous exposure from an infected patient.

35   TRANSMISSION OF BLOOD-BORNE VIRUSES

1   **E – 1 in 30**
       Risk of transmission of 'e' antigen-positive hepatitis B virus is 1 in 3 and
       HIV is 1 in 300.

2**   **N – 6-fold decrease**

3   **C – 1 in 2000**

       See ERN MRCS Book 1, Chapter 2, section 5.6 and Department of
       Health, *Guidance for Clinical Healthcare Workers: Protection against
       Infection with Blood-borne Viruses*, London, Department of Health, 1998.

EMERGENCY MEDICINE AND MANAGEMENT OF TRAUMA

36 THEME: TYPES OF SHOCK

A	Anaphylactic shock
B	Cardiogenic shock
C	Class I haemorrhagic shock
D	Class II haemorrhagic shock
E	Class III haemorrhagic shock
F	Class IV haemorrhagic shock
G	Neurogenic shock
H	Septic shock
I	Spinal shock

From the list above pick the single most appropriate answer for the following clinical scenarios. The items may be used once, more than once or not at all.

1　A 32-year-old man is brought to A&E following a road traffic accident. On arrival, he is anxious and confused, his heart rate is 130 bpm and blood pressure is 90/50 mmHg. Aggressive resuscitation is started. A pelvic fracture is identified on X-ray for which an external fixator is applied. Urine output in the first hour after admission is 10 ml.

2　A 45-year-old man is brought to A&E after being stabbed in the left side of his chest. On arrival, his heart rate is 120 bpm with muffled heart sounds, and his blood pressure is 90/50 mmHg. His neck veins are engorged and air entry is equal bilaterally. His blood pressure fails to improve despite aggressive resuscitation.

3　A 28-year-old motorcyclist is brought into A&E after a high-velocity road traffic accident. On arrival, he is lethargic and his heart rate is 142 bpm with a blood pressure of 88/48 mmHg. His respiratory rate is 36 breaths/min.

36   TYPES OF SHOCK

1**   **E – Class III haemorrhagic shock**

2   **B – Cardiogenic shock**
There is cardiac tamponade secondary to penetrating trauma.

3   **F – Class IV haemorrhagic shock**

*   See ERN MRCS Book 1, Chapter 5, section 2.2 and ATLS student course manual.

*   Haemorrhagic shock:

    *   Class I: heart rate < 100 bpm, normal BP
    *   Class II: heart rate > 100 bpm, normal BP
    *   Class III: heart rate > 120 bpm but < 140 bpm, low BP, confused patient
    *   Class IV: heart rate > 140 bpm and low BP, lethargic patient.

37 THEME: CHOICE OF FLUID FOR RESUSCITATION

A   20 ml/kg bolus of crystalloid solution
B   40 ml/kg bolus of crystalloid solution
C   Cross-matched blood
D   Maintenance crystalloids
E   O negative blood
F   O positive blood
G   Two litres bolus of colloid solution
H   Two litres bolus of 5% dextrose
I   Two litres bolus of normal saline
J   Two litres bolus of Ringer's lactate
K   Type-specific blood

From the list above pick the single most appropriate next step in management for the following clinical scenarios. The items may be used once, more than once or not at all.

1   A 37-year-old man is brought to A&E after sustaining an open fracture of his right tibia. On arrival, his Glasgow Coma Scale (GCS) score is 15/15, blood pressure is 110/70 mmHg and heart rate is 118 bpm.

2   A 6-year-old child is brought to A&E after falling from a first floor window. On examination, airway and breathing are normal. He is tachycardic and hypotensive. GCS score is 15/15.

3   A 40-year-old woman is involved in a road traffic accident and brought to A&E. On examination, her heart rate is 146 bpm, blood pressure is 90/70 mmHg and respiratory rate is 36 breaths/min. Clinically, there are obvious lower limb fractures and her abdomen is distended. A bolus of crystalloid is given with minimal improvement of her haemodynamic parameters.

37   CHOICE OF FLUID FOR RESUSCITATION

1   J – Two litre bolus of Ringer's lactate

2**   A – 20 ml/kg bolus of crystalloid solution

3   E – O negative blood
       Class IV shock and no response to crystalloid resuscitation.

- See ERN MRCS Book 1, Chapter 5, section 2.2 and ATLS student course manual.

- Ringer's lactate is the fluid of choice. If unavailable use normal saline.

- Blood also needs to be added in Class III or IV haemorrhagic shock or when there is a lack of response to crystalloid resuscitation.

- Blood availability time: O negative blood – immediate; type-specific – 10 minutes; cross-matched blood – up to 1 hour.

- Infusion rates in children: crystalloid – 20 ml/kg bolus (may be repeated ×2); packed red cells 10 ml/kg bolus.

38 THEME: TRIAGE

A	Immediate treatment
B	Delayed treatment
C	Treat life-threatening and multisystem injuries first
D	Treat patients with greatest chance of survival first
E	Urgent treatment

From the list above pick the single most appropriate answer for the following clinical scenarios. The items may be used once, more than once or not at all.

1   You are on call when you hear of a bomb blast at a nearby sporting event. You are informed that your hospital will be receiving in excess of 50 seriously injured patients, many of whom have life-threatening injuries. There are problems imitating the 'major incident plan', and when the casualties begin arriving there are only four doctors and six nurses and a medical student available.

2   While on call in a busy district general hospital, you receive two trauma calls simultaneously. There are four doctors split into two teams. The patient whom your team has received has a tension pneumothorax, requiring a needle thoracostomy. The second team is establishing a definitive airway in a second patient. A third patient arrives, who has been triaged 'yellow'.

3   You are the doctor in a rapid response team called to the site of a train derailment. On arrival you see one derailed coach. Most of the passengers have walked away uninjured. In all there are nine passengers who have sustained significant injuries. Six ambulances arrive on the scene. There are two hospitals within a 7 km (5 mile) distance.

38 TRIAGE

1   D – Treat patients with greatest chance of survival first

2   E – Urgent treatment

3**   C – Treat life-threatening and multisystem injuries first

•   See ERN MRCS Book 1, Chapter 5, section 1.4 and ATLS student course manual.

•   In mass casualty treat patients with greatest chance of survival first. In multiple casualties treat life-threatening injury first.

•   Triage involving 'colour coding' of casualties is as follows: green – minor; yellow – delayed; red – immediate; black – deceased.

39 THEME: INITIAL ASSESSMENT OF THE TRAUMA PATIENT

A   Apply direct pressure
B   Apply tourniquet
C   Cervical spine immobilisation
D   Chest drain insertion
E   CT scan of head
F   Limb elevation
G   Nasotracheal intubation
H   Needle cricothyroidotomy
I   Needle thoracostomy
J   Oropharyngeal airway
K   Orotracheal intubation
L   Pericardiocentesis
M   Remove foreign body
N   Seal wound on chest
O   Tracheostomy

From the list above pick the single most appropriate next step in management for the following clinical scenarios. The items may be used once, more than once or not at all.

☐ 1   A 22-year-old man is brought to A&E with severe craniofacial injuries following a road traffic accident. On examination, his heart rate is 92 bpm, blood pressure is 110/70 mmHg and GCS score is 12/15. Air entry is equal bilaterally and his oxygen saturation drops from 92% to 80%. His nostrils and mouth are filled with blood clots and debris that are not cleared with vigorous suction.

☐ 2   A 48-year-old woman is brought to A&E after being involved in a road traffic accident. On examination, the trachea is shifted to the left side and the neck veins are engorged. Her heart rate is 120 bpm and her blood pressure is 90/50 mmHg. There is no air entry on the right side of the chest.

☐ 3   A 32-year-old man is brought to A&E after a fall from a height. On arrival, his heart rate is 120 bpm, blood pressure is 90/50 mmHg and oxygen saturations are 80% on 15 l via a mask with reservoir bag. The neck veins are collapsed. Further examination of his chest reveals dullness on percussion and absent breath sounds, affecting the right hemithorax.

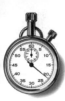

1**   **H – Needle cricothyroidotomy**
This is indicated for upper airway obstruction.

2   **I – Needle thoracostomy**
This is indicated for tension pneumothorax.

3   **D – Chest drain insertion**
This is indicated when there is clinical evidence of (significant) haemothorax.

- See ERN MRCS Book 1, Chapter 5 section 3 and ATLS student course manual.

- According to the ATLS guidelines, the primary survey involves assessment and treatment of ABCDE.

- This is a dynamic process that must be repeated in the trauma room, so that each component is regularly reassessed to detect deterioration.

- Always intervene to ensure that function is restored to normal *before* moving on to the next phase of the primary survey.

40 THEME: ASSESSMENT AND RESUSCITATION OF THE UNCONSCIOUS PATIENT

A   Abdominal X-ray
B   Arterial blood gas analysis
C   Capillary glucose
D   Chest X-ray
E   CT scan of abdomen
F   CT scan of head
G   ECG
H   Intravenous administration of naloxone
I   Rewarming
J   Serum toxicology

From the list above pick the single most appropriate next step in management for the following clinical scenarios. The items may be used once, more than once or not at all.

☐ 1   A 30-year-old man is brought to A&E after being found collapsed at home. On arrival, his GCS score is 7/15 and he is intubated. His pupils are equal bilaterally and reacting to light. His heart rate is 52 bpm and blood pressure is 140/90 mmHg. Capillary glucose and blood gases are within normal limits.

☐ 2   A 48-year-old woman with type I diabetes mellitus is brought to A&E with altered level of consciousness. He husband says that she has been unwell for the past couple of days with a chest infection. She has been vomiting and complaining of abdominal pain for the past few hours. On examination, her heart rate is 110 bpm and her blood pressure is 110/70 mmHg. She is clinically dehydrated. Capillary glucose is 30 mmol and ECG is within normal limits.

☐ 3   You are called to review a 78-year-old woman on the orthopaedic ward who has become increasingly drowsy following a total knee replacement earlier that day. Her heart rate is 68 bpm, her blood pressure is 100/80 mmHg and her oxygen saturations are 80%. You notice that she has a PCA line. You decide to insert an oropharyngeal airway and commence oxygen therapy via a non-rebreathing mask. Examination reveals pinpoint pupils bilaterally.

40 ASSESSMENT AND RESUSCITATION OF THE UNCONSCIOUS PATIENT

1   **F – CT scan of head**
There is a suggestion of raised intracranial pressure (↓ pulse; ↑ BP).

2**   **B – Arterial blood gas analysis**
There is possible ketoacidosis.

3   **H – Intravenous administration of naloxone**
Required for opioid 'overdose'.

See ERN MRCS Book 1, Chapter 5, section 4.2, ATLS student course manual and NICE, *Head injury: triage, assessment, investigation and early management of head injury in infants, children and adults,* London: NICE, 2003 (www.nice.org.uk/page.aspx?o=CG004).

- Unconscious patients can present with a wide range of underlying pathological abnormalities.

- It is crucial to eliminate hypoglycaemia, hypothermia, drugs and toxins as potential (immediately reversible) causes.

- In the post-operative patient opioid toxicity should always be excluded.

41 THEME: CERVICAL SPINE IMAGING IN PATIENTS WITH HEAD INJURY

A	CT scan of the cervical spine	D	Test range of movements of the
B	CT scan and X-ray of the cervical		cervical spine
	spine	E	Three view plain cervical spine
C	Imaging of the cervical spine *not*		X-ray
	indicated at present	F	Two view plain cervical spine X-ray

From the list above pick the single most appropriate course of action in each of the following clinical scenarios. The items may be used once, more than once or not at all.

☐ 1 A 68-year-old woman falls from the top of the stairs at home and lands at the bottom. Her GCS score is 15/15 and all vital parameters are within normal limits. She has a small laceration on her forehead and is complaining of 'slight pain in her neck'. Her neck is immobilised in a hard collar.

☐ 2 A 34-year-old man is brought to A&E following a road traffic accident where he sustained severe head injuries. He has a GCS score of 7/15 and is intubated. His neck is immobilised in a collar. X-ray of his cervical spine is inadequate. He is due to be transferred for a CT scan of his head.

☐ 3 A 42-year-old car driver is brought to A&E after being hit by a large truck. He was drowsy on the scene and his neck was immobilised in a collar. On examination, his GCS score is 15/15 and his vital signs are stable.

42 THEME: MANAGEMENT OF TRAUMATIC WOUNDS

A	Administer anti-tetanus immuno-	D	Exploration
	globulin and tetanus toxoid	E	Exploration and debridement
B	Administer tetanus toxoid	F	Exploration ± joint irrigation
C	Debridement	G	Fasciotomy

From the list above pick the single most appropriate next step in the management for the following clinical scenarios. The items may be used once, more than once or not at all.

☐ 1 A 43-year-old man presents to A&E with a ragged laceration of his right calf after he was stabbed with a broken bottle during a fight on his farm a day ago. On examination, there is soil and devitalised tissue in the wound. The wound is debrided, left open and he is prescribed antibiotics. He is unsure whether he has been vaccinated with tetanus.

☐ 2 A 22-year-old man presents to A&E with an injury to his right middle finger sustained while punching someone on the face during a fight. On examination, there is a puncture laceration over the metacarpophalangeal joint of the middle finger, the depth of which could *not* be accurately assessed.

☐ 3 A 52-year-old man is shot in his left arm during a fight in a pub. On arrival in A&E, his vital signs are stable. There is an entry wound in the anterior aspect of the arm and an exit wound posteriorly.

41 CERVICAL SPINE IMAGING IN PATIENTS WITH HEAD INJURY

1   **E – Three view plain cervical spine X-ray**
Indicated due to pain at rest.

2   **A – CT scan of the cervical spine**
No clinical assessment possible/inadequate radiological assessment.

3**   **E – Three view plain cervical spine X-ray**
Required due to mechanism of injury.

• See ERN MRCS Book 1, Chapter 5, section 3.1 and ATLS student course manual and NICE, *Head injury: triage, assessment, investigation and early management of head injury in infants, children and adults*, London: NICE, 2003 (www.nice.org.uk/page.aspx?o=CG004).

• Assessment of the cervical spine is clinical (when safe!) and radiological.

• All three views (anteroposterior (AP), lateral and open mouth) are necessary to rule out cervical spine fractures.

• CT of the cervical spine can be carried out concomitantly with other CT scans, especially when the plain films are inadequate.

42 MANAGEMENT OF TRAUMATIC WOUNDS

1   **A – Administer anti-tetanus immunoglobulin and tetanus toxoid**

2**   **F – Exploration ± joint irrigation**

3   **D – Exploration and debridement**

• See ERN MRCS Book 1, Chapter 5, section 4.1.

• All patients with tetanus prone wounds (> 6 hours, signs of infection, debris and devitalised tissue, etc.) should receive tetanus toxoid and antitetanus immunoglobulin if they have not been adequately immunised before (three doses of toxoid within 10 years).

• Wounds over joints in the hand need exploration and if found to be penetrating the joint will need irrigation. Failure to do so may result in septic arthritis and loss of function.

• Most gunshot wounds need to be explored and debrided.

43 THEME: USE OF TOURNIQUET IN THE EMERGENCY SETTING

A	Constriction band may be applied	E	Ischaemic gangrene
B	Myoglobinuria	F	Nerve palsy
C	Incomplete arterial occlusion	G	Tourniquet may be applied
D	Incomplete venous occlusion	H	Tourniquet should *not* be applied

From the list above select the single most appropriate answer for the following clinical scenarios. The items may be used once, more than once or not at all.

1 A 22-year-old man sustains a severe traumatic laceration to the right mid-thigh. The paramedic crew arrive at the scene in 15 minutes and find a drowsy man with signs of severe haemorrhagic shock. He has a large wound affecting the thigh with obvious spurting from an artery. Despite application of a 'high-thigh' arterial tourniquet, the bleeding increases.

2 A 48-year-old man is bitten by a snake on the leg while exploring the Australian desert. His friend who is with him recognises that the snake is poisonous. The nearest hospital is 70 km (50 miles) away.

3 A 22-year-old soldier sustains a shrapnel injury to his left thigh. He is bleeding torrentially from a wound in his left thigh and is at risk of exsanguination. Immediate transfer to hospital is not possible.

44 THEME: ACUTE LOSS OF VISION

A	Acute glaucoma	G	Occipital stroke
B	Amaurosis fugax	H	Optic neuritis
C	Central retinal artery occlusion	I	Orbital cellulitis
D	Central retinal vein occlusion	J	Retinal detachment
E	Endophthalmitis	K	Temporal arteritis
F	Migraine	L	Vitreous haemorrhage

From the list above pick the single most appropriate diagnosis for the following clinical scenarios. The items may be used once, more than once or not at all.

1 A 37-year-old man with myopia and a history of floaters in the left eye for the past 2 days presents to the ophthalmic emergency department with sudden loss of vision in his left eye.

2 A 58-year-old woman presents to A&E with a history of sudden loss of vision in her left eye. She also complains of headache, fever, jaw pain and malaise for the past 2 days.

3 A 63-year-old woman with a history of uncontrolled hypertension presents to A&E with a rapidly fading vision in her right eye which she describes as 'a curtain coming down'.

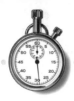

43 USE OF TOURNIQUET IN THE EMERGENCY SETTING

1 **C – Incomplete arterial occlusion**
Venous congestion increases venous pressure and increases 'back-bleeding'.

2** **A – Constriction band may be applied**

3 **G – Tourniquet may be applied**

- The philosophy guiding the use of tourniquets in the emergency setting is that one must be ready to sacrifice the limb to save life.

- Although common in combat situations where there are numerous casualties, their use should be avoided wherever possible.

- In the case of poisonous snake bites, constriction bands to occlude only the superficial veins can be used to reduce systemic absorption of the venom if medical facilities are not available nearby.

44 ACUTE LOSS OF VISION

1** **J – Retinal detachment**
This is more common in patients with myopia.

2 **K – Temporal arteritis**
Urgent temporal artery biopsy to confirm the diagnosis and high dose steroids are indicated to prevent irreversible loss of vision.

3 **B – Amaurosis fugax**
Usually due to thromboembolic events secondary to ipsilateral internal carotid artery stenosis.

See ERN MRCS Book 2, Chapter 3, section 8.3.

PRINCIPLES OF SURGICAL ONCOLOGY

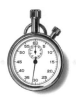

45   THEME: CANCER INCIDENCE AND MORTALITY

A   Bladder cancer
B   Bowel cancer
C   Breast cancer
D   Lung cancer
E   Melanoma
F   Non-melanoma skin cancer (NMSC)
G   Prostate cancer
H   Skin cancer

From the list above select the single most likely diagnosis in each of the scenarios described below. The items may be used once, more than once or not at all.

☐ 1   The leading cause of cancer deaths in men in the UK.

☐ 2   The leading cause of cancer deaths in women in the UK.

☐ 3   The most frequently diagnosed cancer in men in the UK.

☐ 4   The most frequently diagnosed cancer in women in the UK.

46   THEME: BREAST CANCER SCREENING

A   0%
B   1%
C   10%
D   45%
E   75%
F   90%
G   99%
H   100%

From the list above select the most appropriate percentage for each of the scenarios described below. The items may be used once, more than once or not at all.

☐ 1   What proportion of 50–64 year olds take up the UK breast cancer screening programme?

☐ 2   On the breast surgery ward round you are asked by your consultant, 'What has been the increase in the incidence of breast cancer from 1983 to 2002?'

☐ 3   A 55-year-old woman who has been newly diagnosed with breast cancer asks you how likely she is to survive 5 years with current best practice in the UK.

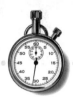

45   CANCER INCIDENCE AND MORTALITY

1   **G – Prostate cancer**

2**   **D – Lung cancer**
This replaced breast cancer in 1999.

3   **F – Non-melanoma skin cancer (NMSC)**

4   **F – Non-melanoma skin cancer (NMSC)**

- See ERN MRCS Book 1, Chapter 3, section 1.4 and Cancer Research UK (http://info.cancerresearchuk.org:8000/cancerstats/) for up-to-date epidemiological data.

- Non-melanoma skin cancer is the commonest cancer diagnosed in men, women and overall in the UK.

- Cancer incidence (excluding NMSC):
    - overall: breast, lung, bowel, prostate
    - men: prostate, lung, bowel, bladder
    - women: breast, bowel, lung, ovarian.

- Cancer mortality:
    - overall: lung, bowel, breast, prostate
    - men: lung, prostate, bowel, oesophagus
    - women: lung, breast, bowel, ovarian.

46   BREAST CANCER SCREENING

1   **E – 75%**

2**   **D – 45%**

3   **E – 75%**

- See ERN MRCS Book 1, Chapter 3, section 1.3 and Cancer Research UK (http://info.cancerresearchuk.org:8000/cancerstats/types/breast/?a=5441) for up-to-date epidemiological data.

- There was an increase in the diagnosis of breast cancer of 45% between 1983 and 2002. Some of this was a transient increase due to screening. The persistent rise is due to other factors.

- The National Health Service Breast Screening Programme (NHSBSP) was introduced in 1986.

- Three-yearly mammography is offered to women aged 50–64 years. Since 2004, this has been extended to include women aged 65–70 years. Women aged over 70 can request mammography once every 3 years, but are not routinely invited.

47 THEME: CHEMOTHERAPEUTIC AGENTS

A	5-Fluorouracil	E	Cyclophosphamide
B	Bacillus Calmette-Guérin (BCG)	F	Herceptin
C	Cisplatin	G	Methotrexate
D	Chlorambucil	H	Tamoxifen

From the list above select the most commonly used chemotherapeutic agents in each of the following scenarios. The items may be used once, more than once or not at all.

☐ 1   A 25-year-old man is diagnosed as having testicular cancer. CT scan of the abdomen and pelvis reveal that the para-aortic lymph nodes are involved.

☐ 2   A 40-year-old woman is diagnosed with breast cancer. Histology shows the tumour to be oestrogen-receptor positive but her-2/neu-receptor negative.

☐ 3   A 60-year-old man is found to have liver metastases following resection of a colorectal cancer thought to be Duke's B at the time of resection.

48 THEME: TUMOUR MARKERS

A	Acid phosphatase
B	Alkaline phosphatase
C	α-Fetoprotein (AFP)
D	β-Human chorionic gonadotrophin (β-hCG)
E	Cancer antigen 125 (CA 125)
F	Carcinoembyonic antigen (CEA)
G	Lactate dehydrogenase (LDH)
H	Prostate-specific antigen (PSA)

From the list above select the tumour marker most likely to be useful in each of the scenarios described below. The items may be used once, more than once or not at all.

☐ 1   A 60-year-old woman is found to have a malignant ovarian neoplasm, which has been completely resected. She is in the clinic for follow up after apparent curative surgery.

☐ 2   A 31-year-old man has an orchidectomy when he is found to have a hard craggy testicular lump. The histology report describes the tumour as a 'purely seminomatous germ cell tumour of the testis'. Which blood test will allow early detection of recurrence in this patient?.

☐ 3   A 70-year-old man has undergone radical radiotherapy for a locally advanced high grade adenocarcinoma of the prostate. There has been an apparent cure based on biochemical testing. What test might have been used to detect this?

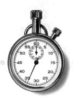

47 CHEMOTHERAPEUTIC AGENTS

1** **C – Cisplatin**
Platinum-based chemotherapy will cure 90% of stages I–III testicular cancer.

2 **H – Tamoxifen**

3 **A – 5-Fluorouracil**
This remains the mainstay of current chemotherapeutic regimens for cancer of the colon.

- See ERN MRCS Book 1, Chapter 3, section 4.3.

- Chemotherapeutic agents may be used to achieve cure, for maintenance of remission or for palliation.

- Adjuvant therapy refers to additional treatment, usually given after surgery where all detectable disease has been removed, but where there remains a statistical risk of relapse due to occult disease.

- Neoadjuvant therapy is given *before* the primary treatment to address 'undetected' (by staging) micrometastases.

- Concomitant chemotherapy refers to administering at the same time as other therapies (eg chemoradiation).

- Herceptin, an antibody directed against her-2/neu is now recommended (by NICE) for oestrogen-receptor-negative tumours that are associated with poor prognosis due to the poor response rate to tamoxifen.

48 TUMOUR MARKERS

1 **E – Ca-125**

2** **G – LDH**

3 **H – PSA**

- See ERN MRCS Book 1, Chapter 3, section 3.5.

- AFP and β-hCG are produced in testicular tumours by trophoblasts and syncytiotrophoblasts, respectively.

- Pure seminomas do not express AFP or β-hCG. However, most seminomas contain an element of trophoblast or syncytiotrophoblast.

- Acid phosphatase monitoring has been superseded by PSA monitoring in prostate cancer treatment.

49 THEME: STAGING OF CANCER

A	A
B	C
C	Ia
D	Ib
E	II
F	IIIa
G	IIIb
H	IVa
I	IVb

From the list above select the correct stage for the tumours described below. The items may be used once, more than once or not at all.

1 A patient has a breast tumour, which is mobile and confined to the breast. There are palpable (mobile) axillary lymph nodes. Your consultant asks you to stage the cancer using the Manchester classification.

2 A patient undergoes resection of an adenocarcinoma of the transverse colon. Histological examination demonstrates invasion through the muscularis mucosa and involvement of lymph nodes. The medical student attached to your firm asks you the Duke's stage of the cancer.

3 A 65-year-old man undergoes a transurethral resection of the prostate (TURP) gland. Prostate cancer is detected in > 5% of the resected tissue during routine histological examination. The patient's son, who is a general practitioner, asks you what the T stage is.

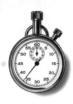

| 49 | STAGING OF CANCER |

1   E – II

2   B – C

3**   D – Ib

- See ERN MRCS Book 1, Chapter 3, section 3.4 and the International Union Against Cancer website (www.uicc.org; go to TNM).

- The appropriate management of a patient with cancer is not possible without knowledge of the extent (stage) of the disease.

- The **TNM** (primary **T**umour, regional lymph **N**odes, distant **M**etastasis) staging system, introduced by the International Union Against Cancer, is becoming the global standard in cancer staging.

- Detection of prostate cancer at TURP is not uncommon, even when it is clinically undetectable. PSA 'screening'-detected prostate cancer is staged T_{1a}. Tumour detectable on digital rectal examination is stage T2.

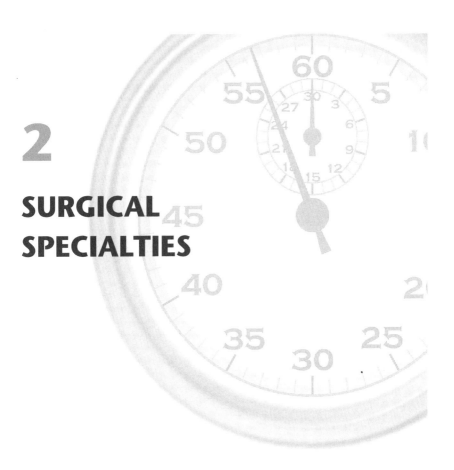

2

SURGICAL
SPECIALTIES

CARDIOTHORACIC SURGERY

50 THEME: THORACIC TRAUMA

A	Aortic dissection
B	Cardiac tamponade
C	Diaphragmatic rupture
D	Flail chest
E	Massive haemothorax
F	Myocardial contusion
G	Oesophageal rupture
H	Pulmonary contusion
I	Simple pneumothorax
J	Tension pneumothorax
K	Tracheobronchial disruption

From the list above pick the single most appropriate diagnosis for the following clinical scenarios. The items may be used once, more than once or not at all.

1 A 28-year-old man is brought to the emergency department having sustained blunt injury to his chest in a road traffic accident. On examination, his pulse rate is 110 bpm, his blood pressure is 80/50 mmHg and his respiratory rate is 30 breaths/min. Further cardiorespiratory examination reveals an elevated jugular venous pressure (JVP), positive Kussmaul's sign and muffled heart sounds on auscultation. Breath sounds are equal on both sides. There are no signs of external haemorrhage.

2 A 43-year-old woman is brought to the emergency department following a road traffic accident. On examination, her heart rate is 118 bpm, her blood pressure is 86/50 mmHg and her respiratory rate is 38 breaths/min. JVP is elevated. The trachea is deviated to the right and the left side of the chest is hyper-resonant to percussion.

3 A 56-year-old cab driver is brought to the emergency department after being involved in a head-on collision with another vehicle at 80 km/h (50 miles/h). He complains of interscapular pain. On examination, his heart rate is 72 bpm, his blood pressure is 110/80 mmHg and his GCS score is 14/15. Chest X-ray shows widened mediastinum.

50 THORACIC TRAUMA

1**   **B – Cardiac tamponade**

2   **J – Tension pneumothorax**

3   **A – Aortic dissection**

- See ERN MRCS Book 1, Chapter 5, section 4.3 and ATLS student course manual.

- Muffled heart sounds and good bilateral air entry in the lungs help differentiate cardiac tamponade from tension pneumothorax.

- Interscapular pain with a widened mediastinum on chest X-ray should raise the suspicion of aortic dissection.

51 THEME: MANAGEMENT OF CHEST TRAUMA

A   Arterial blood gases
B   Arteriography
C   Blood transfusion
D   Chest drain insertion
E   CT scan of the chest
F   Emergency room thoracotomy
G   Intercostal nerve block
H   Intubation and assisted ventilation
I   Needle thoracostomy
J   Chest X-ray
K   Pericardiocentesis

From the list above pick the single most appropriate next course of management for the following clinical scenarios. The items may be used once, more than once or not at all.

☐ **1**   A 33-year-old man is brought to the emergency department after being involved in a road traffic accident. On arrival, his respiratory rate is 40 breaths/min, heart rate is 116 bpm, BP is 90/50 mmHg and the JVP is raised. The trachea is deviated to the right and the left side of the chest is hyper-resonant to percussion. His GCS score is 14/15.

☐ **2**   A 38-year-old woman is brought to the emergency department after sustaining blunt injury to her chest in a road traffic accident. On examination, her pulse rate is 110 bpm, her blood pressure is 80/50 mmHg and her GCS score is 15/15. Her respiratory rate is 30 breaths/min, the percussion note is dull and breath sounds are absent on the right side of chest.

☐ **3**   A 56-year-old construction worker injures the right side of his chest after falling from a height of 9 m (30 feet). On arrival in the emergency department, his GCS score is 13/15, heart rate is 110 bpm, blood pressure is 100/70 mmHg and respiratory rate is 38/min. His GCS score is 13/15. Further examination reveals obvious respiratory distress and a section of his right lateral chest wall moves inward with inspiration. His oxygen saturation drops to 82% despite being administered 100% oxygen via a non-rebreathing mask.

51   MANAGEMENT OF CHEST TRAUMA

1   **I – Needle thoracostomy**
The clinical features of a tension pneumothorax are described. A large bore (14G) needle must be inserted (second intercostal space in the mid-clavicular line).

2**   **D – Chest drain insertion**
The clinical features of a haemothorax are described. This requires formal drainage.

3   **H – Intubation and assisted ventilation**
This patient has a flail segment leading to respiratory compromise.

• See ERN MRCS Book 1, Chapter 5, section 4.3 and ATLS student course manual.

• Immediate decompression (during the primary survey itself) is indicated for the initial treatment of tension pneumothorax. This converts it to a 'simple' pneumothorax that will needed formal tube thoracostomy for definitive treatment.

• The presence of a large flail segment will severely compromise ventilation. Intubation and assisted ventilation is frequently necessary.

52 THEME: PRINCIPLES OF CARDIAC SURGERY

A   DC shock
B   Hypothermia
C   Solution containing magnesium chloride
D   Solution containing potassium chloride
E   Solution containing potassium iodide

From the list above pick the single most appropriate answer for each of the following scenarios. The items may be used once, more than once or not at all.

1   The final year medical student attached to your firm asks you how cardioplegia is most often achieved during open-heart surgery.

2   Following completion of a CABG (carotid artery bypass graft), a patient goes into ventricular fibrillation once they come off bypass and normal perfusion is established. Your boss asks you how this should be managed.

53 THEME: DISORDERS OF THE HEART AND THE GREAT VESSELS

A   Aortic stenosis
B   Atrial septal defect
C   Coarctation of the aorta
D   Eisenmenger's syndrome
E   Mitral stenosis
F   Patent ductus arteriosus
G   Tetralogy of Fallot
H   Total anomalous pulmonary venous drainage
I   Transposition of the great vessels
J   Ventricular septal defect

From the list above pick the single most appropriate diagnosis for the following clinical scenarios. The items may be used once, more than once or not at all.

1   A 25-year-old woman presents to the outpatient clinic with headache, episodes of epistaxis and bilateral leg pain on exercise. On examination, her blood pressure is 170/110 mmHg in both upper limbs. There is a precordial systolic murmur. She has diminished lower limb pulses.

2   An 8-year-old boy attends the outpatient clinic with his mother with history of recurrent respiratory infections and reduced growth. On examination, there is a machinery murmur in the precordium.

3   A 6-year-old girl is referred to the outpatient clinic. Her mother reports episodes when her daughter becomes blue. She also says that she appears to be excessively tired and is smaller than the other children in her class at school. Chest X-ray reveals a boot-shaped heart.

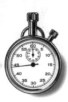

52 PRINCIPLES OF CARDIAC SURGERY

1** D – Solution containing potassium chloride

2 A – DC shock

See ERN MRCS Book 2, Chapter 7, section 1.10.

53 DISORDERS OF THE HEART AND THE GREAT VESSELS

1 C – Coarctation of the aorta

2 F – Patent ductus arteriosus

3** G – Tetralogy of Fallot

- See ERN MRCS Book 2, Chapter 7, section 3.2.

- A difference between upper and lower limb blood pressures in the presence of hypertension and lower limb claudication is diagnostic of coarctation of the aorta.

- Patent ductus arteriosus usually causes minimal symptoms.

- Fallot's tetralogy comprises: ventricular septal defect, pulmonary stenosis, over-riding aorta and right ventricular hypertrophy. Intermittent central cyanosis, squatting episodes and a boot-shaped heart on chest X-ray are classic of this condition.

54 THEME: LUNG CANCER COMPLICATIONS

A   Bony metastasis
B   Brain metastasis
C   Eaton–Lambert syndrome
D   Ectopic adrenocorticotrophic hormone secretion
E   Horner's syndrome
F   Hypercalcaemia
G   Myasthenia gravis
H   Pancoast's syndrome
I   Phrenic nerve palsy
J   Pleural effusion
K   Recurrent laryngeal nerve palsy
L   Superior vena cava obstruction
M   Syndrome of inappropriate antidiuretic hormone secretion (SIADH)

From the list above pick the single most appropriate diagnosis for the following clinical scenarios. The items may be used once, more than once or not at all.

☐ **1** A 65-year-old man receiving chemoradiotherapy for small-cell carcinoma of the lung is brought to the emergency department with seizures. On examination he is drowsy and difficult to arouse. His blood pressure is 160/80 mmHg and heart rate is 74 bpm. He had a CT scan of his brain 2 weeks ago that was normal. His biochemistry results reveal sodium of 110 mmol/l.

☐ **2** A 65-year-old smoker, who was recently diagnosed with squamous cell lung cancer, presents to the clinic with difficulty in breathing. On examination, his face appears bloated and he is extremely dyspnoeic. His conjunctivae are congested and there are distended veins on the chest wall.

☐ **3** A 62-year-old man is being treated for small-cell lung cancer when he presents to the clinic complaining of weakness and fatigue. On examination there is symmetrical, weakness proximal and more prominent in the lower limbs. Muscle strength improves on repetitive use.

54 LUNG CANCER COMPLICATIONS

1	M – SIADH
2	L – Superior vena cava obstruction
3**	C – Eaton–Lambert syndrome

- See ERN MRCS Book 2, Chapter 7, section 4.

- SIADH is a classic paraneoplastic syndrome. The diagnostic features are: low sodium and plasma osmolality in the presence of inappropriately concentrated urine and normal renal/adrenal function.

- Repetitive use improves muscle strength in the Eaton–Lambert syndrome, distinguishing it clinically from myasthenia gravis.

55 THEME: AORTIC DISSECTION

A   Arteriography
B   Blood pressure control
C   Drainage of the clot and repair of the intimal tear
D   No intervention required
E   Serial CT scans of the chest
F   Surgical repair (open graft/endovascular stent)

From the list above pick the single most appropriate management for the following clinical scenarios. The items may be used once, more than once or not at all.

1   A 58-year-old hypertensive man is brought to the emergency department with severe interscapular and central chest pain. On examination, his blood pressure is 150/80 mmHg in the right arm and 110/70 mmHg in the left arm. X-ray of the chest shows a widened mediastinum. A CT scan with contrast demonstrates that the ascending aorta has a false lumen that extends all the way down to the abdominal aorta.

2   A 38-year-old man attends the emergency department with a sudden onset of severe tearing chest and interscapular pain. On examination, his blood pressure is 160/110 mmHg and is equal on both sides. His serum creatinine is 150 μmol/l. Chest X-ray shows widened mediastinum and helical CT with contrast reveals an aortic dissection commencing distal to the origin of the left subclavian artery.

3   A 56-year-old smoker with uncontrolled hypertension presents to the emergency department with a sudden onset of severe interscapular pain while straining in the toilet. On arrival, his blood pressure is 160/110 mmHg. Both femoral pulses are present. His serum creatinine is 99 μmol/l. Helical CT reveals a dissection involving the descending aorta.

55 AORTIC DISSECTION

1   **F – Surgical repair (open graft/endovascular stent)**
This is type-A dissection.

2**   **F – Surgical repair (open graft/endovascular stent)**
This is type-B dissection complicated by renal failure.

3   **B – Blood pressure control**
This is an uncomplicated type-B dissection.

- See ERN MRCS Book 2, Chapter 7, section 5.6.

- There are various classification systems for aortic dissection. The simplest classifies them into type A (involving the ascending aorta) and type B, (does not involve the ascending aorta and often begins distal to the left subclavian artery).

- Type A is associated with high mortality and thus *all* require surgical intervention (open versus endovascular stenting).

- Type B may be complicated by rupture, refractory hypertension, visceral (eg renal failure)/spinal/lower limb ischaemia and severe, chronic pain. The presence of any of these is an indication for surgical intervention.

- In the absence of such complications (uncomplicated type B), management is conservative and concentrates on blood pressure control (vasodilators/β-blockers).

56 THEME: DISEASES OF THE PLEURA

A	Benign pleural effusion
B	Chylothorax
C	Closed pneumothorax
D	Empyema
E	Haemothorax
F	Malignant pleural effusion
G	Mesothelioma
H	Open pneumothorax

From the list above pick the single most appropriate diagnosis for the following clinical scenarios. The items may be used once, more than once or not at all.

1 A 63-year-old smoker presents to the outpatient clinic with gradually worsening shortness of breath. He also complains of loss of weight and appetite. On examination, the right hemithorax is dull to percussion and breath sounds are reduced.

2 A 75-year-old man with stage IV non-Hodgkin's lymphoma with mediastinal lymph node involvement presents to the emergency department with history of worsening shortness of breath. On examination, there is reduced air entry on the left side and percussion note is dull. Aspiration reveals a creamy, opalescent fluid that appears sterile on microscopy.

3 A 36-year-old woman presents to the emergency department with a 4-day history of fever with chills, cough and shortness of breath. On examination, she is febrile and there is reduced air entry in the right lung base with tenderness on percussion.

56   DISEASES OF THE PLEURA

1   **F – Malignant pleural effusion**

2**   **B – Chylothorax**

3   **D – Empyema**

- See ERN MRCS Book 2, Chapter 7, sections 5.2 and 5.3.

- Chylothorax can be due to thoracic duct obstruction or direct injury following surgical procedures. The fluid contains lymphocytes and is sterile.

- Management of empyema involves control of sepsis, drainage of pus and obliteration of the empyema cavity.

57 THEME: COMPLICATIONS OF THORACIC OPERATIONS

A	Acute renal failure	H	Pericardial tamponade
B	Atrial fibrillation	I	Persistent air leak
C	Bleeding	J	Pleural effusion
D	Bronchopleural fistula	K	Pneumonia
E	Congestive cardiac failure	L	Pulmonary embolism
F	Empyema thoracis	M	Subphrenic abscess
G	Myocardial infarction	N	Urinary tract infection

From the list above pick the single most appropriate diagnosis for the following clinical scenarios. The items may be used once, more than once or not at all.

1 A 53-year-old man underwent an oesophagogastrectomy for a carcinoma of the lower third of the oesophagus. On the fourth post-operative day his blood pressure drops to 100/70 mmHg. On examination, he is tachypnoeic and $S_a(O)_2$ is 86% on 4 litres of O_2/min. Arterial blood gases reveal a $p_a(O_2)$ of 8.1 kPa, and a $p_a(CO_2)$ of 2.9 kPa.

2 A 58-year-old man has a pneumonectomy for carcinoma of his right lung. Six days following the procedure, he develops high fever and develops a cough, productive of copious amounts of offensive fluid. Chest X-ray reveals an air-fluid level in the right side of the chest.

3 A 35-year-old woman is brought to the recovery after undergoing a mitral valve replacement. You are called by the recovery nurse as her blood pressure has dropped. On examination, the JVP is elevated, the heart sounds are muffled and there is evidence of pulsus paradox.

57   COMPLICATIONS OF THORACIC OPERATIONS

1   **L – Pulmonary embolism**
Arterial blood gases confirm hyperventilation due to ventilation-perfusion mismatch.

2**   **D – Bronchopleural fistula**

3   **H – Pericardial tamponade**

- Bronchopleural fistula is a serious complication of pneumonectomy with a high mortality rate.

- Cardiac tamponade can occur in the immediate post-operative period following cardiac surgery and demands immediate surgical decompression.

GENERAL SURGERY

THE ABDOMEN

58 THEME: MANAGEMENT OF ABDOMINAL TRAUMA

A   Computed tomography (CT) scan
B   Diagnostic peritoneal lavage (DPL)
C   Focused assessment with sonography for trauma (FAST) scan
D   Immediate laparotomy
E   Observation
F   Repeated clinical examination

From the list above pick the single most appropriate next step in management for the following clinical scenarios. The items may be used once, more than once or not at all.

1   A 32-year-old man is brought to the emergency department after being hit on the left side of the trunk with a baseball bat in a pub brawl. He complains of severe left-sided abdominal pain. On examination his Glasgow Coma Scale (GCS) score is 15/15, his heart rate is 108 bpm and his blood pressure is 110/80 mmHg. Air entry is equal on both sides. Examination of the abdomen reveals left upper quadrant tenderness. Chest X-ray as part of the trauma series reveals lower rib fractures on the left.

2   An 18-year-old man is brought to the emergency department having sustained two stab injuries to the abdomen. On arrival his GCS score is 13/15, his heart rate is 120 bpm and his blood pressure is 68/56 mmHg. Examination of his abdomen revealed bleeding knife wounds in the right hypochondrium. There are no other obvious injuries.

3   A 38-year-old pedestrian is brought to the emergency department after being hit by a car at 80 km/h (50 mph). He was found unconscious and was intubated on the scene by paramedics. His heart rate is 120 bpm and his blood pressure is 90/50 mmHg. He has multiple limb fractures. X-rays of the cervical spine, chest and pelvis are normal. His vital signs fail to improve despite adequate resuscitation.

58   MANAGEMENT OF ABDOMINAL TRAUMA

1   C – FAST scan

2   D – Immediate laparotomy

3**   B – DPL

- See ERN MRCS Book 1, Chapter 5, section 4.4 and ATLS student course manual.

- Stable patient – FAST negative proceed to CT.

- Stable patient – FAST positive proceed to laparotomy/CT if conservative treatment planned.

- Unstable patient and isolated injury – proceed straight to laparotomy.

- Unstable patient and multiple injuries – DPL.

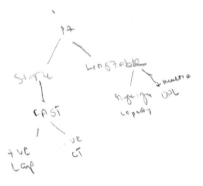

59 THEME: MANAGEMENT OF THE ACUTE ABDOMEN

A	Abdominal ultrasound scan
B	CT scan of the abdomen
C	Diagnostic laparoscopy
D	Electrocardiogram (ECG)
E	Erect chest X-ray
F	Exploratory laparotomy
G	Intravenous antibiotics
H	Urgent Endoscopic retrograde cholangiopancreatography(ERCP)

From the list above pick the single most appropriate next step in management for each of the following clinical scenarios. The items may be used once, more than once or not at all.

☐ 1 A 58-year-old woman with a known history of gallstones presents to the emergency department with epigastric pain radiating to the back. Blood tests on admission reveal haemoglobin 134 g/l (13.4 g/dl), white cell count (WCC) 22 000 cells/mm³, alkaline phosphatase 350 IU/l, aspartate amino-transferase 650 IU/l, corrected calcium 1.9 mmol/l and serum amylase 1100 IU/l. Her blood gases reveal a $p_A(O_2)$ of 9.2 kPa with a base deficit of –5.3. She was admitted to the high-dependency unit (HDU) and managed with fluid resuscitation and invasive monitoring. Forty-eight hours following the admission her physiological compromise remains unchanged.

☐ 2 A 43-year-old man is brought to the emergency department with a 2-day history of pain beginning in the epigastric region, which now involves the entire abdomen. On examination he is dehydrated. His heart rate is 110 bpm and his blood pressure is 90/70 mmHg. Abdominal examination reveals a tender abdomen with generalised guarding and rigidity. Chest X-ray reveals a pneumoperitoneum.

☐ 3 A 60-year-old cab driver is brought to the emergency department with sudden-onset epigastric pain radiating to the left arm. On examination, he is sweating profusely with a heart rate of 55 bpm and a blood pressure of 100/80 mmHg.

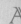

59   MANAGEMENT OF THE ACUTE ABDOMEN

1   **H – Urgent ERCP**
Indicated in gallstone pancreatitis to relieve ampullary obstruction if the patient fails to improve within 48 hours.

2**   **F – Exploratory laparotomy**
Hollow viscus perforation is invariably managed with laparotomy.

3   **D – ECG**
An inferior wall myocardial infarction presentation can mimic acute abdomen.

See ERN MRCS Book 2, Chapter 1, sections 6.1 and 6.2.

60 THEME: RIGHT ILIAC FOSSA PAIN

A	Acute appendicitis
B	Carcinoma of the caecum
C	Crohn's disease
D	Cystitis
E	Diverticulitis
F	Irritable bowel syndrome
G	Mesenteric adenitis
H	Mittelschmerz
I	Pelvic inflammatory disease
J	Rectus sheath haematoma
K	Ruptured ectopic pregnancy
L	Ureteric colic
M	Torsion of ovary

From the list above pick the single most appropriate diagnosis for each of the following clinical scenarios. The items may be used once, more than once or not at all.

☐ 1　A 21-year-old woman is brought to the emergency department with severe pain in the right iliac fossa, referred to the right shoulder. On examination, she is pale, cold and clammy. She has a heart rate of 110 bpm and a blood pressure of 90/70 mmHg. Abdominal examination revealed diffuse tenderness and guarding throughout the lower abdomen.

☐ 2　An 11-year-old girl is brought to the emergency department with a 2-day history of right-sided abdominal pain, fever and vomiting. On examination, she has a temperature of 37.6 °C and a heart rate of 112 bpm. Abdominal examination reveals tenderness in the right iliac fossa.

☐ 3　A 36-year-old woman presents to the emergency department with sudden onset of pain in the right iliac fossa that awoke her from sleep. She does not have any urinary symptoms or discharge per vaginam. On examination, she is in distress. She is afebrile, her heart rate is 120 bpm and there is marked tenderness and guarding in the right iliac fossa. Her last menstrual period was 2 weeks ago. Urine examination is negative for β-human chomonic gonadotrophin (β-hCG), blood and leucocytes.

60   RIGHT ILIAC FOSSA PAIN

1   **K – Ruptured ectopic pregnancy**
Signs of hypovolaemic (haemorrhagic) shock are described. The shoulder pain reflects diaphragmatic irritation from intraperitoneal blood.

2   **A – Acute appendicitis**

3**   **M – Torsion of ovary**
This is characterised by sudden onset of pain. Signs of peritonism are usually evident.

- See ERN MRCS Book 2, Chapter 1, sections 6.1 and 6.2.

- Pregnancy, and its complications, must be excluded in all women of childbearing age presenting with lower abdominal pain.

- Ovarian cyst accidents (torsion/rupture/haemorrhage) may result in lower abdominal pain. In the case of ovarian torsion, the woman is characteristically unwell, often with tachycardia and signs of peritonism. It is more likely to occur in association with ovarian cysts (usually > 5 cm in diameter). As with gonadal torsion in men, prompt diagnosis and emergency surgical intervention (both via laparoscopy) is required to save the gonad.

61 THEME: MANAGEMENT OF LEFT ILIAC FOSSA PAIN

A   Barium enema
B   CT scan of the abdomen and pelvis
C   Diagnostic laparoscopy
D   Flexible sigmoidoscopy
E   Intravenous urogram (IVU)
F   Ultrasound scan of the abdomen
G   Urgent laparotomy

From the list above pick the single most appropriate next step in management for each of the following clinical scenarios. The items may be used once, more than once or not at all.

1   A 68-year-old man with a know history of diverticular disease is brought to the emergency department with fever and pain in the left lower abdomen. Examination of the abdomen revealed tenderness and a suggestion of a mass in the left iliac fossa. His white cell count is 16 000 cells/mm^3.

2   A 32-year-old bus driver presents to the emergency department with acute onset of intermittent left iliac fossa pain radiating to the groin. On examination he is afebrile. There is mild tenderness in the left iliac fossa. Urine dipstick test shows haematuria. His pain does not respond to routine analgesics.

3   A 32-year-old woman presents with a 2-day acute exacerbation of chronic left iliac fossa pain. There is no history of vaginal discharge. Her blood tests and pelvic ultrasound findings are within normal limits.

61 MANAGEMENT OF LEFT ILIAC FOSSA PAIN

1   B – CT abdomen

2   E – IVU

3**   C – Diagnostic laparoscopy

- See ERN MRCS Book 2, Chapter 1, sections 6.1 and 6.2.

- CT scan confirms the diagnosis of diverticulitis and is able to differentiate uncomplicated from complicated (inflammatory mass/abscess/perforation/fistula) diverticular disease.

- Pain and haematuria raises the suspicion of renal tract calculi. Calculi may be evident on the control KUB (kidney ureter bladder) and obstruction can be determined following administration of intravenous contrast.

- Contrary to popular belief (of gynaecology senior house officers (SHOs)!), a normal pelvic ultrasound scan does NOT exclude all potential gynaecological causes of lower abdominal pain (eg uncomplicated endometriosis, pelvic inflammatory disease, ovarian torsion or ovarian cyst accidents). Diagnostic laparoscopy is the gold standard for definitive diagnosis.

62 THEME: ABDOMINAL MASSES 1

A	Abdominal aortic aneurysm	G	Metastatic disease of the liver
B	Carcinoma of the head of pancreas	H	Mucocoele of the gall bladder
C	Carcinoma of the stomach	I	Polycystic kidney disease
D	Divarication of the rectus	J	Pseudocyst of the pancreas
	abdominis muscles	K	Renal cell carcinoma
E	Empyema of gallbladder	L	Splenomegaly
F	Mesenteric cyst		

From the list above pick the single most appropriate diagnosis for the following clinical scenarios. The items may be used once, more than once or not at all.

1 A 70-year-old man presents to the outpatient clinic with 2-month history of severe weight loss followed by jaundice and pruritus for the past 2 weeks. On examination, he looks emaciated. Examination of the abdomen reveals a globular mass in the right hypochondrium that moves with respiration.

2 A 33-year-old man presents to the outpatient clinic with a 6-month history of dull ache in both loins. His blood pressure is 160/100 mmHg. Examination of the abdomen reveals an irregular mass in the right hypochondrium and lumbar region, which does not move with respiration.

3 A 56-year-old alcoholic presents to the outpatient clinic with a 3-week history of swelling in the upper abdomen. He does not have any symptoms related to this apart from slight feeling of pressure in the upper abdomen. One month previously, he was hospitalised for 10 days for severe upper abdominal pain. On examination, there is a smooth mass in the epigastrium.

63 THEME: ABDOMINAL MASSES 2

A	Appendicular mass	E	Diverticular mass
B	Carcinoma of caecum	F	Ovarian cyst
C	Carcinoma of sigmoid colon	G	Psoas abscess
D	Crohn's disease	H	Uterine fibroid

From the list above pick the single most appropriate diagnosis for the following clinical scenarios. The items may be used once, more than once or not at all.

1 A 22-year-old university student presents to the outpatient clinic with a 6-month history of intermittent right iliac fossa pain and increased bowel frequency. She also reports losing 6 kg in weight during the same period. Examination of the abdomen reveals a tender mass in the right iliac fossa.

2 A 60-year-old man presents to the emergency department with a 3-day history of pain in the left lower abdomen and loose stools. On examination, he is febrile and there is a vague tender mass in the left iliac fossa.

3 A 24-year-old woman presents to the outpatient department with chronic right iliac fossa pain. On examination, there is a firm non-tender mass in the right iliac fossa, arising from the pelvis.

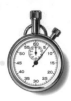

62   ABDOMINAL MASSES 1

1**   B – Carcinoma of the head of the pancreas

2   I – Polycystic kidney

3   J – Pseudocyst of the pancreas

- See ERN MRCS Book 2, Chapter 1, section 8.1.

- According to Courvoisier's law, carcinoma of the head of the pancreas causes dilatation of the 'normal' gallbladder, which becomes palpable.

- Polycystic kidney usually presents during the third/fourth decades and is characterised by abdominal/loin pain, hypertension and bilateral masses.

- Pancreatic pseudocysts usually present after an episode of acute pancreatitis. Non-infected pseudocysts are detectable as a painless mass in the epigastrium.

63   ABDOMINAL MASSES 2

1   D – Crohn's disease

2**   E – Diverticular mass

3   F – Ovarian cyst

- See ERN MRCS Book 2, Chapter 1, section 8.1.

- Abdominal pain, weight loss and loose stools in a young adult should raise the suspicion of inflammatory bowel disease. The presence of a mass is more likely to be due to ileo-caecal Crohn's disease.

- By contrast, such symptoms in older individuals tend to reflect either a colorectal neoplasm or a diverticular mass, the latter being more likely in the presence of raised inflammatory parameters.

- Large ovarian neoplasms, extending out of the pelvis may be detected on abdominal palpation. Pelvic ultrasound is required to differentiate from uterine pathology, and it can help distinguish benign and malignant lesions.

64 THEME: CHRONIC ABDOMINAL PAIN

A   Adhesions
B   Chronic cholecystitis
C   Chronic constipation
D   Chronic pancreatitis
E   Diverticular disease
F   Endometriosis
G   Irritable bowel syndrome
H   Lumbar spine degeneration
I   Ovarian cyst
J   Peptic ulcer disease
K   Pelvic inflammatory disease

From the list above pick the single most appropriate diagnosis for the following clinical scenarios. The items may be used once, more than once or not at all.

1   A 32-year-old man presents to the outpatient clinic with a 4-year history of intermittent colicky, central abdominal pain. He opens his bowels daily and the pain is not affected by defaecation. Five years ago he underwent a laparotomy for multiple stab injuries to his abdomen. Examination of the abdomen reveals a midline scar but is otherwise unremarkable.

2   A 38-year-old woman presents to the outpatient clinic with a 1-year history of intermittent lower abdominal pain relieved by defaecation. She also reports change in bowel habits with alternating constipation and diarrhoea. Abdominal examination is unremarkable. Blood tests and colonoscopy are within normal limits.

3   A 46-year-old man presents to the outpatient clinic with a 2-year history of recurrent epigastric and back pain. He also suffers from weight loss and loose stools, and has recently been diagnosed with diabetes mellitus. Abdominal examination is unremarkable.

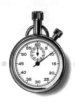

64 CHRONIC ABDOMINAL PAIN

1	A – Adhesions
2	G – Irritable bowel syndrome
3**	D – Chronic pancreatitis

- See ERN MRCS Book 2, Chapter 1.

- The aetiology of pain in patients with post-operative adhesions is ill understood but may reflect recurrent episodes of subacute bowel obstruction/bowel dysfunction.

- Organic pathology *must* be excluded prior to making this diagnosis. Even then it should only be diagnosed when two of the following are present: (i) improvement of pain with defaecation; (ii) onset of abdominal pain is associated with a change in the form of stool; and (iii) the frequency of stools (Longstreth GF, Thompson WG, Chey WD et al. Functional bowel disorders. *Gastroenterology* 2006; 130: 1480–1491).

- Chronic pancreatitis results in hormonal (diabetes) and digestive (steatorrhoea) insufficiency and is characterised by recurrent attacks of abdominal pain.

65   THEME: GASTROINTESTINAL OBSTRUCTION: AETIOLOGY

A   Adhesions
B   Carcinoma of caecum
C   Caecal volvulus
D   Crohn's disease
E   Congenital bands
F   Gallstone ileus
G   Gastric outlet obstruction
H   Hypertrophic pylorus
I   Impacted faeces
J   Intussusception
K   Ischaemic stricture
L   Obstructed hernia
M   Pseudo-obstruction
N   Rectal carcinoma
O   Sigmoid volvulus
P   Superior mesenteric artery syndrome

From the list above pick the single most appropriate diagnosis for the following clinical scenarios. The items may be used once, more than once or not at all.

1   A 55-year-old obese man is brought to the emergency department with a 2-day history of abdominal distension, pain and vomiting. On examination, he is dehydrated, the abdomen is distended and tympanic to percussion and auscultation reveals borborygmi. Examination of the right groin reveals a diffuse swelling.

2   A 66-year-old man presents to the emergency department with a 1-day history of gross abdominal distension, absolute constipation and pain in the left iliac fossa. On examination, he is distressed, the abdomen is grossly distended and there is tenderness and guarding in the left iliac fossa. Plain X-ray of the abdomen reveals the 'coffee bean' sign.

3   A 20-year-old woman presents to the outpatient clinic with a 6-week history of epigastric pain, early satiety and bile-stained vomiting. Three months ago she was hospitalised for 4 weeks following a road traffic accident in which she sustained multiple injuries. During this episode she lost almost a third of her weight. Abdominal examination reveals a succussion splash.

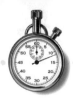

65 GASTROINTESTINAL OBSTRUCTION: AETIOLOGY

1   **L – Obstructed hernia**

2   **O – Sigmoid volvulus**

3**   **P – Superior mesenteric artery syndrome**

- See ERN MRCS Book 2, Chapter 1, section 6.3.

- Meticulous inspection of the hernial orifices should be conducted in patients with bowel obstruction.

- The coffee bean sign is characteristic of a sigmoid volvulus.

- Features of the superior mesenteric artery syndrome are bile-stained vomiting, pain relieved on lying prone or on the left side along with a recent history of weight loss.

66 THEME: GASTROINTESTINAL OBSTRUCTION: INVESTIGATION AND MANAGEMENT

A   Abdominal ultrasound
B   Abdominal X-ray
C   Adhesiolysis
D   Barium follow through
E   Barium swallow
F   Colonoscopy
G   CT scan of the abdomen
H   Hartmann's procedure
I   Oesophagogastroduodenoscopy
J   Resection and primary anastomosis
K   Sigmoidoscopy and flatus tube insertion
L   Water-soluble contrast enema

From the list above pick the single most appropriate next step in management for the following clinical scenarios. The items may be used once, more than once or not at all.

1   A 72-year-old debilitated woman who has been hospitalised under the care of the medical team for 2 weeks for pneumonia has a 3-day history of abdominal distension, pain, vomiting and absolute constipation. On examination, the abdomen is grossly distended and tympanic and bowel sounds are absent. Plain X-ray of the abdomen reveals colonic dilatation involving the caecum, and the ascending and transverse colon.

2   A 4-week-old baby boy is brought to the emergency department by his mother with a 3-day history of projectile vomiting. On examination, he is dehydrated and peristalsis is visible in the epigastrium.

3   A 68-year-old Afro-Caribbean woman presents to the emergency department with severe generalised abdominal pain, following a 6-day history of absolute constipation. On examination, her heart rate is 110 bpm and her blood pressure is 100/70 mmHg. The abdomen is grossly distended and peritonitic. A plain abdominal X-ray reveals a closed loop large bowel obstruction with Rigler's sign. At laparotomy, there is a perforated, obstructed sigmoid neoplasm with gross faecal contamination of the peritoneal cavity.

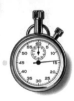

66 GASTROINTESTINAL OBSTRUCTION: INVESTIGATION AND MANAGEMENT

1   **L – Water-soluble contrast enema**

2   **A – Abdominal ultrasound**

3   **H – Hartmann's procedure**

- See ERN MRCS Book 2, Chapter 1, section 6.3.

- A water-soluble single contrast enema is necessary to exclude organic obstruction in patients with suspected pseudo-obstruction.

- A hypertrophic pyloric canal can be detected by ultrasound scan.

- Rigler's sign, also known as the double wall sign, is seen on abdominal X-ray when air is present on both sides of the intestine (ie in pneumoperitoneum).

- Hartmann's procedure (Henri Albert Hartmann) involves rectosigmoid resection with permanent colostomy. The proximal end of the distal segment is oversewn and left in place leaving a blind rectal pouch.

67 THEME: MANAGEMENT OF ABDOMINAL SEPSIS

A   Abdominal ultrasound
B   Colonoscopy
C   Intravenous antibiotics
D   Laparotomy
E   Leucocyte scan
F   Radiological drainage
G   Splenectomy
H   Transrectal drainage

From the list above pick the single most appropriate next step in management of the following clinical scenarios. The items may be used once, more than once or not at all.

☐ **1** A 29-year-old man presents to the emergency department with a 1-week history of fever, lassitude, anorexia and weight loss. Three weeks prior to this, he was operated for a perforated duodenal ulcer. On examination, he is febrile and there is evidence of small pleural effusion on the right side. A full blood count shows leucocytosis and a chest X-ray reveals an elevated right dome of the diaphragm.

☐ **2** A 67-year-old man with known history of diverticular disease presents to the emergency department with a 2-day history of left lower abdominal pain and constipation. On examination he is febrile and there is tenderness and guarding in the left iliac fossa. Abdominal ultrasound reveals a large abscess adjacent to the sigmoid colon.

☐ **3** A 20-year-old man presents to the emergency department with a 5-day history of fever, loose stools and tenesmus. He was discharged from hospital 2 weeks ago after an appendicectomy for a perforated appendix. On examination he is febrile; rectal examination revealed a boggy mass anteriorly. CT of the pelvis confirms the diagnosis.

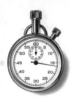

67 MANAGEMENT OF ABDOMINAL SEPSIS

1	F – Radiological drainage
2	F – Radiological drainage
3**	H – Transrectal drainage

- See ERN MRCS Book 2, Chapter 1, section 6.4.

- Radiological drainage is the treatment of choice for subphrenic abscess and paracolic abscess whenever feasible.

- Transrectal drainage under general anaesthesia is the treatment of choice to drain large pelvic abscesses, such as those complicating appendicectomy.

68 THEME: GROIN SWELLINGS

A	Ectopic testes
B	Encysted hydrocele of the cord
C	Femoral artery aneurysm
D	Femoral hernia
E	Inguinal hernia
F	Inguinal lymphadenopathy
G	Lipoma
H	Pseudoaneurysm
I	Psoas abscess
J	Saphena varix
K	Sarcoma

From the list above pick the single most appropriate diagnosis for the following clinical scenarios. The items may be used once, more than once or not at all.

1 A 48-year-old woman presents to the outpatient clinic with a 1-year history of a lump in the right groin. On examination, the lump is above and medial to the pubic tubercle. There is an expansile impulse on coughing and the lump reduces spontaneously on lying down.

2 A 56-year-old woman presents to the outpatient clinic with a 3-month history of a pigmented lesion (mole) on her right shin that has been increasing in size. She also complains of weight loss. Examination of the groin reveals three firm round swellings below the inguinal ligament.

3 A 43-year-old immigrant presents to the emergency department with back pain, fever, nights sweats and a lump in his left groin. On examination, there is tenderness in the thoracolumbar spine. Abdominal examination reveals fullness in the left iliac fossa and a fluctuant swelling in the femoral triangle. There is a cough impulse and cross fluctuation can be elicited.

68 GROIN SWELLINGS

1   E – Inguinal hernia

2   F – Inguinal lymphadenopathy

3**   I – Psoas abscess

- See ERN MRCS Book 2, Chapter 1, section 1.2.

- Inguinal herniae arise above and medial to the pubic tubercle, whereas femoral herniae arise below and lateral to the pubic tubercle.

- Femoral herniae are commoner in women but inguinal herniae remain the commonest herniae in women.

- Malignant melanomas metastasise via the lymphatics to the inguinal nodes. These can be felt as multiple, firm swellings **below** the inguinal ligament.

- The presence of the classic history of tuberculosis (weight loss, night sweats etc) together with back pain suggests spinal tuberculosis. Psoas abscess can sometimes become very large to the extent that 'cross fluctuation' can be elicited while compressing the right iliac fossa swelling.

69   THEME: ABDOMINAL HERNIAE

A   Femoral hernia
B   Incarcerated hernia
C   Incisional hernia
D   Inguinal hernia
E   Maydl's hernia
F   Obstructed hernia
G   Paraumbilical hernia
H   Richter's hernia
I   Sliding hernia
J   Spigelian hernia
K   Strangulated hernia
L   Umbilical hernia

From the list above pick the single most appropriate diagnosis for the following clinical scenarios. The items may be used once, more than once or not at all.

1   A 50-year-old woman presents to the emergency department with a 2-day history of abdominal pain and diarrhoea. Abdominal examination reveals mild lower abdominal tenderness. Examination of the groin revealed a tender irreducible swelling below the inguinal ligament and lateral to the pubic tubercle.

2   A 45-year-old man presents to the emergency department with a 24-hour history of central abdominal pain, abdominal distension and absolute constipation. On examination, he is dehydrated and tachycardic. Examination of the abdomen reveals central distension and increased bowel sounds. Examination of the groin revealed an irreducible, non-tender swelling in the left groin.

3   A 56-year-old man presents to the outpatient clinic with a 6-month history of a swelling below the umbilicus on the left side. On examination, there is a swelling 3 cm below and lateral to the umbilicus. There is a positive cough impulse and the swelling reduces spontaneously on lying down.

69 ABDOMINAL HERNIAE

1   H – Richter's hernia

2   F – Obstructed hernia

3**   J – Spigelian hernia

- See ERN MRCS Book 2, Chapter 1, section 1.2.

- Richter's hernia is due to strangulation of part of the bowel; symptoms may mimic gastroenteritis until total obstruction occurs.

- Obstructed herniae are associated with features of bowel obstruction (abdominal pain and distension, vomiting and constipation).

- Strangulation is associated with erythema and tenderness, often with systemic signs (tachycardia).

- Spigelian herniation is an acquired ventral hernia through the linea semilunaris.

70 THEME: INTESTINAL FISTULAE

A	Barium enema
B	Barium follow through
C	Cystoscopy
D	CT-guided drainage
E	Fistulogram
F	Intravenous antibiotics
G	Intravenous fluids
H	Laparotomy
I	Loop stoma
J	Octreotide
K	Oesophagogastroduodenoscopy
L	Oral contrast study
M	Total parenteral nutrition

From the list above pick the single, most appropriate management for the following clinical scenarios. The items may be used once, more than once or not at all.

1 A 38-year-old man has been in the intensive care unit (ICU) for the past 3 weeks after undergoing surgery for necrotising pancreatitis. While on the unit, the nursing staff report a clear discharge from a small opening in his laparotomy wound. The total output from the fistula is 300 ml/day. He is receiving supplementary fluids and his electrolytes are within normal limits.

2 A 63-year-old woman presents to the outpatient clinic with 3-month history of intermittent left-sided abdominal pain. She was otherwise fit and well. A barium enema is arranged, following which the patient attends A&E, reporting passage of white urine.

3 A 22-year-old woman with a history of Crohn's disease presents to the emergency department with a 2-day history of right-sided abdominal pain and a faeculent discharge from a wound in the right lower abdomen. Examination of the abdomen reveals a vague tender mass in the right iliac fossa. CT scan of the abdomen reveals a 10 × 5 cm abscess in the right iliac fossa.

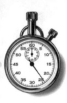

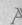

70   INTESTINAL FISTULAE

1**   **J – Octreotide**

2   **C – Cystoscopy**

3   **D – CT-guided drainage**

- See ERN MRCS Book 2, Chapter 1, section 7.3.

- Initial treatment of fistulae includes resuscitation, elimination of sepsis and nutritional support. Then delineation of the fistula and definitive management can be planned.

- Octreotide may help in reducing output from fistulae and aid healing.

- Colovesical fistulae may complicate diverticular disease.

- Enteroenteral and enterocutaneous fistulae may complicate Crohn's disease.

71 THEME: GASTROINTESTINAL STOMAS

A	Appendicostomy	G	Loop ileostomy
B	Caecostomy	H	No stoma
C	End colostomy	I	Open gastrostomy
D	End ileostomy	J	Percutaneous endoscopic
E	Feeding jejunostomy		gastrostomy (PEG)
F	Loop colostomy		

From the list above pick the single most appropriate stoma for the following clinical scenarios. The items may be used once, more than once or not at all.

☐ 1   A 45-year-old man with a history of ulcerative pancolitis refractory to medical treatment undergoes a restorative proctocolectomy.

☐ 2   A 12-year-old girl presents with severe, disabling, intractable constipation. She underwent Duhamel's procedure for Hirschsprung's disease during the first month of life. She has failed to respond to maximal medical therapy for her constipation. Her surgeon suggests a procedure to allow irrigation of the colon to facilitate emptying.

☐ 3   A 62-year-old woman is recovering from a brainstem stroke she has 3 weeks ago. She is unable to swallow and is losing weight rapidly.

72 THEME: COMPLICATIONS OF SPLENECTOMY

A	Atelectasis	G	Pancreatic fistula
B	Deep vein thrombosis	H	Pancreatic pseudocyst
C	Gastric perforation	I	Portal vein thrombosis
D	Gastric stasis	J	Pulmonary embolism
E	Lower lobe pneumonia	K	Splenosis
F	Overwhelming post-splenectomy sepsis (OPSS)	L	Subphrenic abscess

From the list above pick the single most appropriate diagnosis for the following clinical scenarios. The items may be used once, more than once or not at all.

☐ 1   A 12-year-old boy is brought to A&E by his parents with a 3-day history of high fever and a cough productive of rusty coloured sputum. On examination, he is flushed and temperature is 39.5 °C. He underwent splenectomy 18-months ago following a road traffic accident.

☐ 2   A 23-year-old woman had a laparoscopic splenectomy for auto-immune haemolytic anaemia. She was discharged on day 7 post-operatively. The next day she is found collapsed at home and is brought to A&E. She is hypotensive and hypoxic.

☐ 3   A 56-year-old woman presents to A&E 10 days following a splenectomy with fever and pleuritic chest pain. Examination of the chest reveals dullness to percussion and reduced air entry in the left base. Examination of the abdomen reveals tenderness in the left hypochondrium.

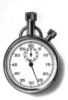

71 GASTROINTESTINAL STOMAS

1   G – Loop ileostomy

2**   A – Appendicostomy

3   J – PEG

* See ERN MRCS Book 2, Chapter 1, section 6.5.

* Restorative proctocolectomy involves resection of the entire colon and rectum and creation of an ileal pouch. A temporary loop ileostomy to divert faecal stream is usually constructed.

* Malone's antegrade continence enema (ACE or MACE) involves the creation of an appendicostomy in the right iliac fossa using Mitrofanoff's principle to provide a non-refluxing channel that may be intermittently catheterised to perform antegrade washout of the colon and rectum. It can be employed for the treatment of faecal soiling secondary to anorectal anomalies or severe paediatric constipation.

* PEG is indicated in neurological diseases with impaired swallowing in a patient with an intact and functional gastrointestinal tract.

72 COMPLICATIONS OF SPLENECTOMY

1**   F – OPSS

2   J – Pulmonary embolism

3   L – Subphrenic abscess

* See ERN MRCS Book 2, Chapter 1, section 4.11.

* OPSS is caused by encapsulated organisms (*Pneumococcus*, *Meningococcus* and *Haemophilus influenzae*). Prophylaxis is with penicillin and polyvalent vaccines.

* A subphrenic abscess may be associated with a 'sympathetic' pleural effusion.

UPPER GASTROINTESTINAL SURGERY

73 THEME: DYSPHAGIA

A   Achalasia
B   Anxiety
C   Benign stricture
D   Bronchial carcinoma
E   Carcinoma of the oesophagus
F   Diffuse oesophageal spasm
G   Foreign body
H   Goitre
I   Neurological disorder
J   Oesophageal candidiasis
K   Oesophageal perforation
L   Pharyngeal pouch
M   Plummer–Vinson syndrome
N   Reflux oesophagitis
O   Scleroderma

For each of the following clinical scenarios, select the single most appropriate diagnosis from the list above. The items may be used once, more than once or not at all.

☐ 1 A 39-year-old man reports progressive difficulty swallowing solids and now also liquids occurring over a period of 18–24 months. Clinical examination is unremarkable.

☐ 2 A 34-year-old woman presents with a 6-month history of difficulty swallowing solids. A barium swallow and an upper gastrointestinal endoscopy fail to identify any abnormalities. There is evidence of high amplitude and prolonged contractions on oesophageal manometry.

☐ 3 A 41-year-old woman reports a 12-month history of difficulty swallowing associated with retrosternal chest pain and nocturnal coughing and vomiting. Clinical examination is unremarkable.

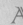

73 DYSPHAGIA

1 **C – Benign stricture**
Slow progression and lack of 'alarm' features provide clues to the diagnosis.

2** **F – Diffuse oesophageal spasm**
Exclusion of organic disease suggests oesophageal dysmotility.

3 **N – Reflux oesophagitis**

• See ERN MRCS Book 2, Chapter 1, sections 2.2–2.6.

• Dysphagia is difficulty swallowing. Odynophagia is pain on swallowing.

• Causes of dysphagia can be classified as:

  – intrinsic oesophageal disorders (organic and functional)
  – extrinsic oesophageal disorders (compression in the neck/mediastinum)
  – generalised disorders (usually neurological).

• Dysphagia at any age is one of the referral criteria for 'suspected upper gastrointestinal cancer' and should prompt urgent referral by general practitioners.

• The investigation of choice is upper gastrointestinal endoscopy. Additional investigations, depending on likely/actual cause, include barium swallow, manometry, pH studies, CT scan.

74 THEME: OESOPHAGEAL CARCINOMA

A   Barium swallow
B   Chest X-ray
C   CT scan of chest and abdomen
D   Curative surgical resection (oesophagectomy)
E   History and clinical examination
F   Oesophageal manometry
G   Palliative (non-surgical) therapy
H   pH studies
I   Staging laparoscopy
J   Upper gastrointestinal endoscopy and biopsy

For each of the following clinical scenarios, select the single most appropriate next step in management from the list above. The items may be used once, more than once or not at all.

☐ 1   A 78-year-old man presents with a history of weight loss and dysphagia. Examination is unremarkable. Upper gastrointestinal endoscopy and biopsy confirms the presence of an adenocarcinoma at the gastro-oesophageal junction. CT scan suggests the presence of peritoneal disease but no evidence of distant metastasis.

☐ 2   A 54-year-old woman with a history of Barrett's oesophagus presents with worsening dysphagia. Examination is unremarkable and a chest X-ray reveals no obvious abnormalities. Biopsy taken at upper gastrointestinal endoscopy reveals invasive adenocarcinoma.

☐ 3   A 71-year-old man presents with a long-history of weight loss and vomiting. Upper gastrointestinal endoscopy and biopsy confirms the presence of an invasive squamous cell carcinoma. Chest X-ray reveals a left-sided pleural effusion, and a cytology specimen from this yields adenocarcinoma cells.

74 OESOPHAGEAL CARCINOMA

1** **I – Staging laparoscopy**
This is most useful in the assessment of tumours of the gastro-oesophageal junction and when there is suspicion of peritoneal disease.

2 **C – CT scan of chest and abdomen**
The findings of the scan will dictate further management.

3 **G – Palliative (non-surgical) therapy**
Because distant metastases confirmed.

- See ERN MRCS Book 2, Chapter 1, section 2.9 and Allum WH, Griffin SM, Watson A et al, Guidelines for the management of oesophageal and gastric cancer. *Gut* 2002; 50 (Suppl V): v1–v23).

- Accurate staging allows identification of patients who will potentially benefit from curative surgery, and those in whom palliation is appropriate.

- T stage assessed using CT (under-stages) and/or endoscopic ultrasound (better accuracy); N stage assessed using CT (poor sensitivity and specificity), endoscopic ultrasound, laparoscopy; M stage using chest X-ray, CT (MRI/bronchoscopy in selected cases).

- Surgery is only contemplated in fit patients in whom cure is feasible, ie localized tumours ($T_{1,2}$) with no nodal involvement or distant metastases.

- Two-phase Ivor–Lewis oesophagectomy is most frequently employed, which involves preliminary laparotomy then right thoracotomy (left impractical due to aortic arch). Third cervical phase may be necessary in proximal tumours.

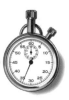

75 THEME: GASTRO-OESOPHAGEAL REFLUX DISEASE (GORD)

A   24-hour pH study
B   Antireflux surgery
C   Barium swallow
D   Chest X-ray
E   CT scan of chest and abdomen
F   H$_2$ antagonists
G   History and clinical examination
H   Oesophageal manometry
I   Oesophageal mucosa biopsy
J   pH studies
K   Proton pump inhibitors (PPIs)
L   Reduce alcohol intake
M   Upper gastrointestinal endoscopy
N   Weight loss

For each of the following clinical scenarios, select the single most appropriate next step in management from the list above. The items may be used once, more than once or not at all.

1   A 48-year-old woman presents with a history of 'heartburn' and reflux of food on bending over. The oesophagus appeared macroscopically normal during upper gastrointestinal endoscopy and biopsy fails to reveal any significant abnormalities. Despite a 3-month trial of PPIs, she remains symptomatic and is demanding that 'something be done'.

2   A 31-year-old ballerina has a history of severe gastro-oesophogeal reflux disease (GORD) with demonstrable severe oesophagitis on upper gastro-intestinal endoscopy. Although clinically very effective in ameliorating her symptoms, she has been unable to tolerate therapy with various PPIs due to gastrointestinal side effects.

3   A 44-year-old woman is referred for an opinion by one of the respiratory physicians. She has been investigated for recurrent episodes of pneumonia, which has proved unrewarding. However, the physician has astutely recorded a history of significant reflux disease and dysphagia. Accordingly, upper gastrointestinal endoscopy was organised, which has confirmed macroscopic and microscopic evidence of uncomplicated oesophagitis.

4   A 27-year-old lawyer presents with daily, troublesome symptoms of heartburn and acid regurgitation, which have not responded to several 'over-the-counter' preparations. The remainder of the clinical history and examination is unremarkable.

75 GASTRO-OESOPHAGEAL REFLUX DISEASE (GORD)

1** **J – pH studies**
No oesophagitis, thus 24-hour pH monitoring is required before contemplating antireflux surgery.

2 **B – Antireflux surgery**
Objective criteria for antireflux surgery met.

3 **B – Antireflux surgery**
Reflux with respiratory complications is an indication for antireflux surgery.

4 **K – Proton pump inhibitors (PPIs)**
Severe symptoms refractory to over-the-counter treatment. No alarm symptoms.

• See ERN MRCS Book 2, Chapter 1, sections 2.3 and 2.4.

• Reflux occurs in asymptomatic individuals, and 20% of patients with endoscopic oesophagitis never have symptoms of reflux.

• Not all patients with typical symptoms of reflux have oesophagitis.

• Thus diagnostic tests facilitate diagnosis but not always necessary if history obvious without alarm symptoms.

• Treatment options include: simple measures (weight loss, avoidance smoking/alcohol etc), medical therapy and surgery.

• PPIs most effective treatment especially for severe symptoms/oesophagitis.

• Antireflux surgery is restricted to those with objective evidence of reflux (erosive oesophagitis/abnormal acid reflux on 24-hour monitoring) and:

  – failure to respond to medical treatment
  – who do not want/tolerate medical treatment (particularly young patients who require years of treatment)
  – develop respiratory complications.

76 THEME: MANAGEMENT OF DYSPEPSIA

A	Barium swallow
B	Chest X-ray
C	CT scan
D	*Helicobacter pylori* eradication therapy
E	*H. pylori* serology
F	History and clinical examination
G	Medical therapy (H$_2$ antagonists or PPIs)
H	Modification of precipitating factors (smoking/alcohol etc)
I	Oesophageal manometry
J	pH studies
K	Routine upper gastrointestinal endoscopy ± biopsy
L	Urgent (< 2 weeks) upper gastrointestinal endoscopy ± biopsy
M	Ultrasound abdomen
N	Withdraw causative medication

For each of the following clinical scenarios, select the single most appropriate next step in management from the list above. The items may be used once, more than once or not at all.

1 A 59-year-old woman presents with a 2-month history of central upper abdominal pain and bloating not relieved by defaecation. There are no 'alarm symptoms' present. Clinical examination is unremarkable.

2 A 41-year-old woman presents with a chronic history of heartburn. There are no 'alarm symptoms' present. Clinical examination is unremarkable. The general practitioner (GP) has sent the result of her *H. pylori* serological examination, which is negative.

3 A 34-year-old male smoker presents with central upper abdominal pain and postprandial vomiting. There are no other associated symptoms. Clinical examination is unremarkable.

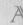

76 MANAGEMENT OF DYSPEPSIA

1 **L – Urgent (< 2 weeks) upper gastrointestinal endoscopy ± biopsy**
New onset in a patient > 55 years old requires urgent investigations, irrespective of presence/absence of alarm symptoms.

2 **G – Medical therapy (H_2 antagonists or PPIs)**
Criteria for investigations not met. As patient is *H. pylori* negative, empirical treatment indicated.

3** **L – Urgent (< 2 weeks) upper gastrointestinal endoscopy ± biopsy**
Such symptoms warrant urgent referral for investigations at any age.

- See ERN MRCS Book 2, Chapter 1, section 3.4 and NICE Clinical Guideline 17. http://www.nice.org.uk/pdf/CGO17NICEguideline.pdf

- Dyspepsia refers to pain or discomfort centred in the upper abdomen.

- Causes essentially include GORD, peptic ulcer disease, non-ulcer (functional) dyspepsia.

- Urgent investigation of dyspepsia is required at any age in patients with:

  - chronic gastrointestinal bleeding
  - dysphagia
  - progressive unintentional weight loss
  - persistent vomiting
  - iron deficiency anaemia
  - epigastric mass
  - suspicious barium meal result.

- Urgent investigation is also required in patients > 55 years old with unexplained and persistent recent-onset dyspepsia alone.

- Recommended management of uninvestigated dyspepsia involves either: (i) empirical treatment with a PPI; or (ii) tests for (C13 urea breath test or lab-based serology) and treatment of *H. pylori* infection.

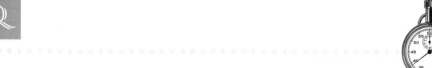

77 THEME: MANAGEMENT OF STOMACH CANCER

A   Barium study
B   CT scan of chest and abdomen
C   Endoscopic ultrasound
D   History and clinical examination
E   Palliative (non-surgical) therapy
F   Partial gastrectomy and lymphadenectomy
G   Routine upper gastrointestinal endoscopy ± biopsy
H   Staging laparoscopy
I   Total gastrectomy and lymphadenectomy
J   Urgent (< 2 weeks) upper gastrointestinal endoscopy ± biopsy
K   Ultrasound scan of abdomen

For each of the following clinical scenarios, select the single most appropriate next step in management from the list above. The items may be used once, more than once or not at all.

☐ 1   A 54-year-old woman is found to have a histological proved bulky adenocarcinoma of the distal third (antrum) of the stomach. Endoscopic ultrasound and CT scan suggest that this is a T_2 lesion with no evidence of lymphatic or distant metastases.

☐ 2   A 71-year-old man presents with a history of dyspepsia and melaena. Clinical examination reveals an epigastric mass, which proves to be a neoplasm of the proximal third of the stomach on CT scan. There is no evidence of nodal or distant metastases.

☐ 3   A 64-year-old man presents with a recent onset of dyspepsia. Upper gastro-intestinal endoscopy confirms the presence of an adenocarcinoma in the proximal third of the stomach. A chest X-ray is unremarkable. CT evaluation of the lesion is limited due to problems distending the stomach during the study, although no distant metastases were evident.

77   MANAGEMENT OF STOMACH CANCER

1   **F – Partial gastrectomy and lymphadenectomy**
        The patient has been adequately staged and has a potentially curable
        lesion.

2   **J – Urgent (< 2 weeks) upper gastrointestinal endoscopy ± biopsy**
        Although clinically likely, cancer has not been proved histologically.

3**   **C – Endoscopic ultrasound**
        This is particularly useful for T staging in this scenario.

•   See ERN MRCS Book 2, Chapter 1, section 3.6 and Allum WH, Griffin
        SM, Watson A et al, Guidelines for the management of oesophageal and
        gastric cancer. *Gut* 2002; 50 (Suppl V): v1–v2.

•   Accurate staging allows identification of patients who will potentially
        benefit from curative surgery, and those in whom palliation is
        appropriate.

•   T stage is best assessed using endoscopic ultrasound, although CT
        provides complementary information; N stage is assessed using CT (poor
        sensitivity and specificity), endoscopic ultrasound, laparoscopy (useful
        when suspicion of peritoneal disease); M stage is usually assessed using
        CT of chest/abdomen.

•   Type of gastrectomy (partial versus total), extent of lymphadenectomy
        (D1, D2, D3) and gastric reconstruction (Bilroth I or II or Roux-en-Y) is
        dictated by location and nature of tumour, and surgeon's choice.

•   Latest guidelines recommend total gastrectomy for proximal/middle-
        third tumours and partial gastrectomy for distal tumours and D1, D2,
        D3 lymphadenectomy for all potentially curable lesions.

78 THEME: COMPLICATIONS OF UPPER GASTROINTESTINAL SURGERY

A	Anastomotic leakage
B	Anastomotic stricture
C	Chronic afferent loop syndrome
D	Chylothorax
E	Diarrhoea
F	Dumping syndrome
G	Early satiety
H	Enterogastric reflux
I	Gastric outlet obstruction (GOO)
J	Haemorrhage
K	Malnutrition
L	Recurrent ulceration
M	Recurrent laryngeal nerve injury
N	Vitamin B_{12} deficiency

For each of the following clinical scenarios, select the single most appropriate surgical complication from the list above. The items may be used once, more than once or not at all.

1 A 59-year-old man undergoes an Ivor–Lewis oesophagectomy for adenocarcinoma of the oesophagus. Although systemically well, the output from the chest drain becomes increasingly cloudy following reintroduction of oral intake.

2 A 41-year-old man presents with a history of persistent epigastric discomfort associated with intermittent vomiting of food mixed with bile within an hour of eating. He previously underwent a partial gastrectomy 12-months ago for a perforated gastric ulcer (benign). On examination he is pale and has a body mass index (BMI) of 19. Full blood count reveals haemoglobin 101 g/l (10.1 g/dl).

3 A 68-year-old woman undergoes an elective subtotal gastrectomy for a proximal third carcinoma. You review her in the outpatient clinic 6 weeks following discharge. She reports palpitations and anxiety at every mealtime. She has also been troubled by postprandial colic and occasional vomiting.

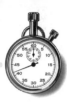

1   **D – Chylothorax**
This presents within 7 days following reintroduction of feeding,
especially fat-containing nutrients. Treatment involves early
re-exploration and ligation.

2**   **H – Enterogastric reflux**
Bile in the vomitus and anaemia (due to 'bilious gastritis') differentiates
this from GOO.

3   **F – Dumping syndrome**
The presence of vasomotor symptoms differentiate this from GOO.

• See ERN MRCS Book 2, Chapter 1, section 3.4.

• As with any operation complications may be early/late or
general/specific to the procedure.

• Specific complications occur due to:

  – anastomotic problems (leakage/stricture/inflammation)
  – vagotomy (diarrhoea/atony)
  – injury to surrounding structures (chylothorax/recurrent laryngeal
    nerve injury/haemorrhage)
  – loss of storage capacity and function (dumping/vitamin
    deficiency/malnutrition).

• Dumping syndrome occurs due to rapid gastric emptying and a
hyperosmolar jejunal load, with resultant massive fluid shifts. Symptoms
are divided into vasomotor (occur towards the end of the meal) and
gastrointestinal (occur later but within 30 minutes of eating).

• Enterogastric reflux is common after gastrectomy. Chronic exposure of
gastric mucosa to intestinal contents leads to gastritis (25% develop
anaemia). Primary or secondary Roux-en-Y reconstruction addresses the
problem.

79 THEME: UPPER GASTROINTESTINAL HAEMORRHAGE

A   Arterial angiogram ± selective embolisation
B   Barium study
C   Discharge from hospital
D   *H. pylori* eradication therapy
E   History and clinical examination
F   Insertion of central line
G   Insertion of two 14G cannulae
H   Insertion of two 18G cannulae
I   Omeprazole 20 mg stat then 2 mg/h infusion
J   Omeprazole 40 mg stat then 4 mg/h infusion
K   Omeprazole 80 mg stat then 8 mg/h infusion
L   Repeat upper gastrointestinal endoscopy
M   Sengstaken–Blakemore tube insertion
N   Surgical intervention
O   Transfer to HDU
P   Upper gastrointestinal endoscopy on next available list
Q   Upper gastrointestinal endoscopy once haemodynamically stable
R   Upper gastrointestinal endoscopy within 24 hours

For each of the following clinical scenarios, select the single most appropriate next step from the list above. The items may be used once, more than once or not at all.

1 A 54-year-old woman presents with fresh haematemesis. She is adequately resuscitated and undergoes urgent upper gastrointestinal endoscopy during which a bleeding duodenal ulcer is successfully injected with adrenaline 1:10 000.

2 A 78-year-old man with a history of emphysema and hypertension is admitted with coffee-ground haematemesis and melaena. His haemoglobin on admission was 80 g/l (8.0 g/dl). Following resuscitation with 4 units of packed red cells he undergoes upper gastrointestinal endoscopy, where a bleeding duodenal is successfully 'clipped'. One day later he has a further episode of haematemesis associated with hypotension. The haemoglobin concentration is 75 g/l (7.5 g/dl). At repeat upper gastrointestinal endoscopy there is a large amount of blood in the stomach, which is obscuring the views in the proximal duodenum.

3 A 72-year-old woman on the orthopaedic ward develops fresh haematemesis following a hemiarthroplasty. She has a past history of congestive cardiac failure, diabetes mellitus and chronic renal impairment. On arrival, her pulse is 105 bpm and BP is 85/50 mmHg. Her haemoglobin concentration is 55 g/l (5.5 g/dl) and clotting screen is normal. You commence full resuscitative measures but despite transfusing 6 units of packed red cells, she has further episodes of hypotension.

4 A 55-year-old man presents with a history of melaena. He has a past history of angina and is receiving treatment for carcinoma of the prostate. On examination his pulse is 85 bpm and blood pressure is 110/75 mmHg. His haemoglobin level is 105 g/l (10.5 g/dl) and a clotting screen is normal.

79　UPPER GASTROINTESTINAL HAEMORRHAGE

1** **K – Omeprazole 80 mg stat then 8 mg/h infusion**
High-dose PPI therapy is indicated once haemostasis is achieved.

2 **N – Surgical intervention**
Indicated as: (i) 1 × rebleed; and (ii) inadequate endoscopy with no haemostasis.

3 **Q – Upper gastrointestinal endoscopy once haemodynamically stable**
This patient has severe upper gastrointestinal haemorrhage and requires endoscopy once stable. Even those likely to require surgery should have varices excluded prior to laparotomy, even if with on-table gastroscopy.

4 **G – Insertion of two 14G cannulae**
Adequate resuscitation is often neglected in patients with upper gastrointestinal haemorrhage. Large-bore (short) cannulae deliver fluids faster than narrow-bore (long) central lines, although the latter may be useful for fluid balance following initial resuscitation.

- See ERN MRCS Book 2, Chapter 1, section 3.5 and Palmer KR, Non-variceal upper gastrointestinal haemorrhage: guidelines. *Gut* 2002; 51 (Suppl IV): iv1–iv6.

- Mortality is 10%. It is highest in elderly people and those with co-morbidities. Paradoxically, surgical intervention must not be delayed in such patients.

- Causes include: peptic ulcer (35–50%), gastroduodenal erosions (8–15%), oesophagitis (5–15%), varices (5–15%), Mallory–Weiss tears (15%) and Carcinoma (1%).

- Management involves: (i) aggressive resuscitation/initial management, (ii) assessment of severity and (iii) definitive management.

- Severity is assessed using scoring systems (eg Rockall), which incorporate age, haemodynamic status, comorbidity and endoscopic findings. High-risk patients are those with increasing age, comorbidity, tachycardia/hypotension and endoscopic stigmata of haemorrhage (clot/bleeding vessel).

- Endoscopy should be undertaken in all patients and may enable haemostasis. If rebleeding occurs, one further attempt at endoscopic haemostasis is acceptable. High-dose PPI infusion reduces rebleed rates but not mortality.

- Surgical intervention for uncontrolled haemorrhage at endoscopy and 1–2 rebleeds. Options may be limited (under-running/excision) or extensive (partial gastrectomy).

80 THEME: FUNCTIONAL DISORDERS OF THE UPPER GASTROINTESTINAL TRACT

A   Achalasia
B   Aerophagia
C   Chagas' disease
D   Chronic idiopathic intestinal pseudo-obstruction (CIPO)
E   Diffuse oesophageal spasm
F   Functional (non-ulcer) dyspepsia
G   Functional dysphagia
H   Functional vomiting
I   Globus
J   Nutcracker oesophagus
K   Rumination syndrome
L   Visceral hypersensitivity

For each of the following clinical scenarios, select the single most appropriate diagnosis from the list above. The items may be used once, more than once or not at all.

☐ 1 A 54-year-old woman presents with a long history of central upper abdominal pain associated with heartburn. Upper gastrointestinal endoscopy and 24-hour pH studies are normal. A barium study and CT scan are unremarkable.

☐ 2 A 38-year-old teacher presents with a history of dysphagia and retrosternal chest pain. All cardiac investigations and an upper gastrointestinal endoscopy are normal. A barium study and follow through reveals a dilated oesophagus but normal-calibre small intestine.

1   **F – Functional (non-ulcer) dyspepsia**
        These are classic symptoms of dyspepsia but without an organic cause.

2**   **A – Achalasia**
        Oesophageal dilatation occurs in isolation in achalasia and in
        combination with small bowel dilatation in Chagas' disease and CIPO.

- See ERN MRCS Book 2, Chapter 1, section 2.5.

- Functional disorders are characterised by chronic or recurrent
  gastrointestinal symptoms not explained by organic or biochemical
  abnormalities.

- Diagnosis is by exclusion of organic causes.

- Physiological abnormalities of visceral sensory and/or motor function are
  increasingly recognised as important in their aetiology. Tests of
  physiological function are useful in identifying such abnormalities.

- Visceral dilatation is a feature of achalasia, Chagas' disease and CIPO.

- Achalasia is characterised by loss of ganglion cells in the oesophagus
  leading to unco-ordinated peristaltic contractions and failure of
  relaxation of the lower oesophageal sphincter, ultimately leading to
  dilatation. Hypo-/aganglionosis is also evident in Chagas' disease but it
  affects the entire gastrointestinal tract leading to extensive dilatation.

HEPATOBILIARY AND PANCREATIC SURGERY

81 THEME: CAUSES OF JAUNDICE

A   Amyloidosis
B   Biliary atresia
C   Bile duct stricture
D   Carcinoma head of the pancreas
E   Cholangitis
F   Cirrhosis
G   Crigler–Najjar syndrome
H   Dubin–Johnson syndrome
I   Drug-induced hepatitis
J   Gallstones
K   Gilbert's syndrome
L   Haemolytic anaemia
M   Multifactorial jaundice
N   Viral hepatitis

For each of the following clinical scenarios, select the single most appropriate diagnosis from the list above. The items may be used once, more than once or not at all.

1   A 69-year-old retired publican presents with jaundice on a background of several months of severe upper abdominal pain that is unrelated to meals. On examination, he is thin, deeply jaundiced and a mass is palpable in the right upper quadrant (RUQ). Dipstick urinalysis is positive for bilirubin but negative for urobilinogen.

2   A 71-year-old man undergoes an emergency laparotomy for a perforated sigmoid diverticulum with faecal peritonitis. Postoperatively, he is transferred to ICU where he is hypotensive. He is commenced on inotropes, meropenem and metronidazole. On day 2 post operatively, he becomes jaundiced and his blood results reveal a bilirubin concentration of 94 μmol/l, ALP 201 IU/l and aspartate aminotransferase 158 IU/L.

3   A 22-year-old student develops generalised lethargy and arthralgia, with loss of appetite and upper abdominal pain. Concerned about the discoloration of his skin, he presents to A&E where he is found to have bilirubin and urobilinogen on urinalysis. Serum bilirubin is 174 μmol/l, ALP is 180 IU/l and AST is 458 IU/l.

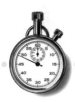

1 **D – Carcinoma head of the pancreas**
Courvoisier's law applies. Urinalysis confirm a post-hepatic cause.

2** **M – Multifactorial jaundice**
Factors include: (i) ↑ bilirubin production (blood transfusion);
(ii) hepatocellular damage (drugs/shock); (iii) cholestasis
(sepsis/shock/drugs).

3 **N – Viral hepatitis**
Typical history with AST disproportionately elevated versus ALP.

• See ERN MRCS Book 2, Chapter 1, section 4.3.

• Haem is broken down into bilirubin (and iron), which is bound to
albumin (unconjugated) and transferred to liver. Here it is conjugated in
the hepatocytes and excreted into the gut where it is converted to
urobilinogen, some of which is absorbed and enters the enterohepatic
circulation and may enter the systemic circulation and be excreted by
the kidneys. The remainder is oxidised to urobilin and excreted in the
stool.

Causes of jaundice and laboratory findings

	Urine	Bilirubin	LFTs
Prehepatic (haemolysis)	↑ urobilinogen	↑ Unconjugated	↑ or →
Hepatic (syndromes/drugs Hepatitis/cirrhosis)	↑ urobilinogen ↑ bilirubin	↑ Conjugated and unconjugated	↑ AST
Post-hepatic (stones/CA)	↑ urobilinogen	↑ Conjugated	↑ ALP

Courvoisier's law states that, in the presence of jaundice, an enlarged
gallbladder is unlikely to be due to gallstones (gallbladder is chronically
fibrosed with stones and cirrhosis and does not dilate); rather carcinoma
of the pancreas or the lower biliary tree is more likely (normal
gallbladder that distends due to distal bile duct obstruction).

82 THEME: MANAGEMENT OF THE JAUNDICED PATIENT

A   Administration of fresh frozen plasma (FFP)
B   Administration of im vitamin K 10 mg
C   Administration of iv vitamin K 10 mg
D   Administration of po vitamin K 10 mg
E   Check serum amylase
F   Commence broad-spectrum antibiotics (after relevant cultures taken)
G   Encourage oral fluid intake
H   Hepatitis serology
I   Insertion of urinary catheter
J   Intravenous fluid resuscitation
K   Laparoscopic cholecystectomy
L   Liver biopsy
M   Re-check coagulation screen
N   Re-check LFTs
O   Transfer to HDU
P   Urgent abdominal ultrasound
Q   Urgent ERCP
R   Urgent magnetic resonance cholangiopancreatography (MRCP)

For each of the following clinical scenarios, select the single most appropriate next step in management from the list above. The items may be used once, more than once or not at all.

☐ 1   A 49-year-old woman who is on the waiting list for laparoscopic cholecys-tectomy presents with a 2-day history of RUQ pain, associated with uncon-trollable shivering. On examination she is pyrexial, deeply jaundiced and tender in the RUQ but haemodynamically stable. Her blood tests reveal a bilirubin concentration of 150 μmol/l, an ALP of 401 IU/l and an AST of 203 IU/l, a normal amylase and an international normalised ratio (INR) of 1.1. You commence fluid resuscitation and antibiotics and monitor her urine output hourly. The next morning, she remains pyrexial and an ultrasound reveals multiple stones in the gallbladder and a common bile duct (CBD) diameter of 10 mm.

☐ 2   A 71-year-old man is admitted with obstructive jaundice secondary to gallstones. Appropriate fluid resuscitation has provoked a decent urine output. His latest blood results are improving slightly, revealing a bilirubin concentration of 80 μmol/l, an ALP of 501 IU/l, an AST of 78 IU/l and an international normalised ratio (INR) of 2.1. He is awaiting an MRCP.

☐ 3   A 42-year-old woman presents with a 2-day history of upper abdominal pain and vomiting. On direct questioning, she reports dark urine. On examina-tion she is apyrexial and mildly jaundiced. She is tender across the upper abdomen. Urinalysis is negative. Blood investigations sent by the A&E sister reveal a bilirubin of 45 μmol/l, an ALP of 200 IU/l, an AST is 45 IU/l and an INR of 1.0. An intravenous fluid infusion of crystalloid is in progress.

1   Q – Urgent ERCP
Clinical evidence of cholangitis (pain, jaundice, rigors). The bile duct obstruction needs to be relieved **as soon as possible.**

2** C – Administration of iv vitamin K 10 mg
Evidence of coagulopathy due to failure absorption of (fat-soluble) vitamin K dependent factors (II, VII, IX, X). Not absorbed after po (the current problem!); im may lead to haematomata when coagulopathic. No fresh frozen plasma (FFP) yet as no bleeding/planned intervention

3   E – Check serum amylase
Exclusion of acute pancreatitis is the priority at this point, as missing this diagnosis and delaying appropriate treatment is potentially disastrous.

• See ERN MRCS Book 2, Chapter 1, sections 4.3 and 5.

• Definitive treatment directed at cause.

• Management is supportive and includes prevention/aggressive treatment of:

  – Hepatorenal syndrome. Treatment: aggressive fluid resuscitation, fluid balance monitoring (hourly via catheter in deep jaundice), ?CVP, ensure polyuric, daily U&Es.
  – Sepsis due to stasis secondary to biliary obstruction. Treatment: monitor for pyrexia, cultures if pyrexia, prompt/high dose antibiotics, prompt relief of obstruction (ERCP).
  – Coagulopathy. Treatment: monitor INR, prophylaxis/aggressive correction with vitamin K iv FFP prior to ERCP/surgery.
  – Pancreatitis (gallstones commonest cause of obstructive jaundice and pancreatitis thus they may co-exist!). Treatment: monitor clinically, check serum amylase/lipase, aggressive treatment if develops, consideration of prompt ERCP in severe cases.

83 THEME: DISORDERS OF THE BILIARY SYSTEM

A	Acalculus cholecystitis
B	Acute cholangitis
C	Acute cholecystitis
D	Biliary stricture
E	Carcinoma of the gallbladder
F	Cholangiocarcinoma
G	Chronic cholecystitis
H	Gallstones
I	Empyema of the gallbladder
J	Primary biliary cirrhosis
K	Primary sclerosing cholangitis

For each of the following clinical scenarios, select the single most appropriate diagnosis from the list above. The items may be used once, more than once or not at all.

1 A 50-year-old long-standing sufferer of ulcerative colitis attends the out-patient clinic with a 6-month history of weight loss and generalised pruritus. He is clinically jaundiced with a bilirubin concentration of 94 μmol/l and an elevated ALP of 250 IU/l. MRCP reveals the presence of multifocal strictures of the intrahepatic and extrahepatic bile ducts.

2 A 32-year-old woman with known gallstones presents with a 36-hour history of RUQ pain and anorexia. On examination there is no evidence of jaundice or pallor. She is pyrexial and tachycardic and Murphy's sign is positive. Her white cell count (WCC) is elevated but all other blood and radiological investigations are normal.

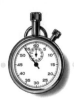

1** K – Primary sclerosing cholangitis

2 C – Acute cholecystitis
Pyrexia and elevated WCC confirm inflammatory process, differentiating from a diagnosis of biliary colic

- See ERN MRCS Book 2, Chapter 1, sections 5.3 and 5.4.

- Gallstones are the commonest disorder of the biliary system, affecting women twice as often as men. Ten per cent of women are affected by their fifth decade.

- Primary sclerosing cholangitis occurs most commonly common in patients with inflammatory bowel disease. Multifocal strictures are diagnostic.

- Primary biliary cirrhosis is a disease characterised by inflammatory destruction of the small bile ducts within the liver, leading to cirrhosis of the liver. Its cause is unknown but it is thought to be an autoimmune disease. About 90% of patients are women. Most commonly, the disease is diagnosed in people between the ages of 40 and 60 years.

84 THEME: COMPLICATIONS OF GALLSTONES

A   Acute cholecystitis
B   Acute pancreatitis
C   Ascending cholangitis
D   Biliary colic
E   Carcinoma of the gallbladder
F   Chronic cholecystitis
G   Gallstone ileus
H   Empyema of gallbladder
I   Mucocoele of gallbladder
J   Obstructive jaundice
K   Perforation of the gallbladder

For each of the following clinical scenarios, select the single most appropriate complication from the list above. The items may be used once, more than once or not at all.

1   A 28-year-old presents with a 12-hour history of RUQ pain referred to the shoulder. She is not clinically jaundiced and is apyrexial. Abdominal examination reveals mild tenderness in the right hypochondrium. All haematological, biochemical and radiological investigations are unremarkable.

2   A 42-year-old woman with known gallstones is admitted with RUQ discomfort. On examination she is apyrexial and not jaundiced. Palpation of the abdomen reveals a non-tender fullness in the right hypochondrium.

3   A 65-year-old diabetic man is admitted with a presumptive diagnosis of acute cholecystitis. Ultrasound of the abdomen reports multiple gallstones in the gallbladder, which is thick-walled. There is no bile duct dilatation. Despite 2 days of conservative therapy, he deteriorates clinically becoming pyrexial, tachycardic and hypotensive. On examination, he has generalised peritonitis. His WCC is elevated but his liver function tests (LFTs) and serum amylase are within normal limits. An arterial blood gas reveals a metabolic acidosis.

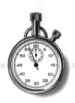

84　COMPLICATIONS OF GALLSTONES

1　**D – Biliary colic**
All inflammatory parameters are normal.

2　**I – Mucocoele of gallbladder**
Gallbladder enlargement in absence of raised inflammatory markers is likely due to mucocoele formation (secondary to a stone in Hartmann's pouch).

3**　**K – Perforation of the gallbladder**
Generalised peritonitis in this situation is either due to a perforation or acute pancreatitis.

- See ERN MRCS Book 2, Chapter 1, section 5.3.

- There are three types of gallstone: cholesterol stones (20%); bile pigment stones (5%); and mixed (75%).

- The majority of gallstones are asymptomatic with only 7% of patients who are initially asymptomatic requiring surgery for complications over the next 5 years.

- The clinical presentations/complications of gallstones is easiest considered anatomically, ie gallbladder (fundus/Hartmann's pouch), cystic duct, CBD, small intestine.

85 THEME: ASSESSMENT OF PATIENTS WITH GALLSTONES

A	Check serum amylase
B	History and clinical examination
C	Laparoscopic cholecystectomy
D	Laparoscopic cholecystectomy with on-table cholangiography
E	Liver biopsy
F	Repeat liver function tests (LFTs)
G	Routine abdominal ultrasound
H	Routine ERCP
I	Routine MRCP
J	Urgent abdominal ultrasound
K	Urgent ERCP
L	Urgent MRCP

From the list above select the single most appropriate next step in the assessment of the patients in each of the following clinical scenarios. The items may be used once, more than once or not at all.

1 A 35-year-old woman was previously admitted with an episode of acute cholecystitis secondary to gallstones when an ultrasound scan excluded the presence of CBD dilatation. Six months later she attends pre-admission clinic for elective laparoscopic cholecystectomy but reports a recent episode of pale stools.

2 A 59-year-old man with gallstones previously demonstrated on ultrasound is admitted with recent onset RUQ pain, pruritus and dark urine. On examination, he is jaundiced but systemically well. Blood investigations reveal a bilirubin concentration of 65 μmol/l, an ALP of 286 IU/l, an AST of 39 IU/l and an INR of 1.0. Serum amylase is normal.

3 A 48-year-old schoolteacher is admitted with severe gallstone pancreatitis. She is mildly jaundiced with a bilirubin of 90 μmol/l. Ultrasound scan suggests the presence of a stone in the distal CBD, which measures 8 mm.

85 ASSESSMENT OF PATIENTS WITH GALLSTONES

1   **F – Repeat liver function tests (LFTs)**
     Possible for stones to have entered CBD since previous ultrasound thus
     check LFTs to ensure normal bilirubin in view of recent pale stools.

2   **J – Urgent abdominal ultrasound**
     This will establish whether there are any stones in/diameter of the CBD.

3** **K – Urgent ERCP**
     Advocated in the management of severe gallstone pancreatitis to
     decompress the CBD

•   See ERN MRCS Book 2, Chapter 1, section 5.3.

•   The aim of investigation is to confirm the diagnosis of gallstones,
     exclude complications and exclude the presence of stones in the CBD.

•   The pattern of abnormal liver enzymes can suggest a diagnosis of
     cholestasis (disproportionately elevated ALP), but abdominal ultrasound
     is the most useful adjunct in diagnosis.

•   MRCP/ERCP is indicated in the presence of: (i) obstructive jaundice; or
     (ii) CBD dilatation (> 5 mm).

•   MRCP is diagnostic; ERCP can be therapeutic.

•   The aim of ERCP is to clear the CBD of stones prior to surgery. As the
     cystic duct is clipped during cholecystectomy, residual stones may result
     in a build-up of pressure in the CBD and hence the cystic duct,
     potentially resulting in displacement of the clips and a bile leak.

86 THEME: MANAGEMENT OF PATIENTS WITH ACUTE PANCREATITIS

A	Check serum amylase
B	Check serum lipase
C	Commence broad-spectrum antibiotics (after relevant cultures taken)
D	Commence enteral nutrition
E	Commence parenteral nutrition
F	CT guided aspiration
G	CT scan of abdomen
H	Encourage oral fluid intake
I	Insertion of a central line for venous pressure monitoring
J	Insertion of urinary catheter for hourly urinary output monitoring
K	Intravenous fluid resuscitation
L	Laparotomy and necrosectomy
M	Maintain 'nil by mouth'
N	Routine abdominal ultrasound
O	Routine ERCP
P	Routine MRCP
Q	Transfer to HDU
R	Transfer to tertiary unit
S	Urgent abdominal ultrasound
T	Urgent ERCP
U	Urgent MRCP

For each of the following clinical scenarios, select the single most appropriate next step in management from the list above. The items may be used once, more than once or not at all.

1 A 49-year-old woman is admitted with upper severe epigastric pain and vomiting. As she has a markedly elevated serum amylase you make a diagnosis of acute pancreatitis. She has a modified Glasgow pancreatitis score of 1 (raised urea). On examination she looks dehydrated and is tachycardic. Aggressive fluid resuscitation with crystalloids has been commenced.

2 A 51-year-old woman is referred by an A&E SHO as she is jaundiced. In addition, she reports a 12-hour of severe epigastric pain.

3 A 29-year-old man was admitted 48 hours ago with a diagnosis of acute pancreatitis. You are asked to review the patient on the ward, as his saturations are 90% on 4 litres of oxygen. Having checked all of the relevant parameters he has a modified Glasgow pancreatitis score of 4.

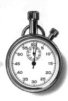

86 MANAGEMENT OF PATIENTS WITH ACUTE PANCREATITIS

1   **J – Insertion of urinary catheter for hourly urinary output monitoring**
First adjunct to assessing fluid balance.

2   **A – Check serum amylase**
It is important not to miss a diagnosis of acute pancreatitis in any patient with abdominal pain.

3**   **Q – Transfer to HDU**
This patient has severe pancreatitis predicted by his Glasgow score and evidenced by respiratory failure (O_2 saturations <90% indicate a $p(O_2) <$ 10 kPa = respiratory failure! Management in an HDU setting is mandatory.

- See ERN MRCS Book 2, Chapter 1, section 5.7 and British Society of Gastroenterology. UK guidelines for the management of acute pancreatitis (*Gut* 2005; 54: 1–9).

- Overall mortality is 5–10%. One quarter develop severe disease with organ failure and mortality rises to 25% in this cohort of patients.

- The initial management of acute pancreatitis involves immediate, aggressive resuscitation and assessment of severity.

- The Atlanta criteria identify **actual** severe disease in the presence of organ dysfunction (eg low $p(O_2)$/elevated creatinine, indicating respiratory and renal dysfunction, respectively) and are increasingly used in preference to Ranson's criteria and the Glasgow scoring system, which only **predict** disease progression.

- Longer-term management comprises: (i) systemic treatment (support of organ systems); and (ii) local treatment (pancreatic necrosis).

87 THEME: COMPLICATIONS OF ACUTE PANCREATITIS

A   Acute renal failure
B   Acute respiratory distress syndrome
C   Chronic pancreatitis
D   Foregut obstruction
E   Haemorrhage
F   Hypovolaemia
G   Infected pancreatic necrosis
H   Multiorgan failure
I   Pancreatic abscess
J   Pancreatic duct stricture
K   Pancreatic necrosis
L   Pseudocyst formation

From the list above, select the single most likely complication in each of the following clinical scenarios. The items may be used once, more than once or not at all.

1   A 72-year-old woman is admitted with severe acute pancreatitis (modified Glasgow score of 4). Her urine output in the past 24 hours is 400 ml. She has a haemoglobin of 115 g/l (11.5 g/dl), a creatinine of 201 μmol/l and is hypoxic with a $p_a(O_2)$ of 7.9 kPa.

2   A 39-year-old alcoholic man is in ICU with organ failure due to severe acute pancreatitis. He is on inotropes, intubated and ventilated and is being fed enterally via a nasogastric tube. His fluid balance for the past 24 hours reads:

In		Out	
Intravenous fluids	4200 ml	Urine output	2100 ml
Inotrope infusion	200 ml	Nasogastric aspirates	1500 ml
Nasogastric tube feed	2160 ml	Vomit	500 ml

3   A 46-year-old man attends the outpatient clinic following a recent admission with acute pancreatitis. He reports intermittent upper abdominal pain and vomiting. On examination there is a large non-tender mass in the epigastrium.

1   **H – Multiorgan failure**
This patient has evidence of respiratory and oliguric renal failure.

2**   **D – Foregut obstruction**
High nasogastric tube aspirates and vomiting confirm foregut
obstruction (secondary to peripancreatic inflammation/oedema causing
extrinsic obstruction).

3   **L – Pseudocyst formation**
Usually requires > 4 weeks from onset of pancreatitis and is often linked
to disruption of the pancreatic duct.

•   See ERN MRCS Book 2, Chapter 1, section 5.7 and British Society of
Gastroenterology. UK guidelines for the management of acute
pancreatitis (*Gut* 2005; 54: 1–9).

•   Complications may be: (i) local affecting the pancreas <pm>
surrounding structures (pancreatic necrosis ± infection, pseudocyst
formation, haemorrhage due to disruption of splenic vessels, foregut
obstruction etc); or (ii) systemic affecting distant organ function.

•   Surgical intervention has become less common with advances in
intensive care. It is reserved for cases of infective pancreatic necrosis,
where necrosectomy may be performed. The high mortality of this
procedure has lead to 'minimally invasive' techniques being employed
to debride, irrigate and drain the retroperitoneum.

88 THEME: MANAGEMENT OF CHRONIC PANCREATITIS

A	Abdominal ultrasound	E	Enzymatic replacement therapy
B	Check random blood glucose	F	Hormonal replacement therapy
C	CT scan of abdomen (with pancreatic protocol)	G	Opioid analgesia
		H	Percutaneous coeliac plexus blockade
D	Endoscopic retrograde cholangiopancreatography	I	Simple analgesia

For each of the following clinical scenarios, select the single most appropriate next step in management from the list above. The items may be used once, more than once or not at all.

1 A 54-year-old man with a diagnosis of chronic pancreatitis attends the outpatient clinic with a new onset of steatorrhoea and weight loss. Random blood glucose is normal.

2 A 66-year-old woman is referred by to the outpatient clinic with severe intermittent epigastric pain and weight loss. She has a history of excess alcohol consumption and has previously been admitted with acute pancreatitis on several occasions. An abdominal ultrasound scan yielded suboptimal views of the pancreas due to 'overlying bowel gas'.

89 THEME: CARCINOMA OF THE PANCREAS

A	Abdominal ultrasound scan	E	Gastrojejunostomy formation
B	CA 19–9 measurement	F	Percutaneous fine-needle aspiration cytology (FNAC)
C	CT scan of abdomen (with pancreatic protocol)	G	Surgical resection (pancreatectomy)
D	ERCP	H	Staging laparoscopy

For each of the following clinical scenarios, select the single most appropriate next step in management from the list above. The items may be used once, more than once or not at all.

1 A 74-year-old man presents with weight loss, epigastric pain and obstructive jaundice. CA 19–9 is 90 U/ml and bilirubin concentration is 165 μmol/l. Ultrasound reveals an obstructing lesion at the head of the pancreas and multiple liver metastases.

2 A 55-year-old man attends outpatients with weight loss and severe abdominal pain, which is referred to the back. CA 19–9 is 10 U/ml and an ultrasound scan has revealed a heterogeneous mass in the tail of the pancreas of unknown aetiology.

3 A 64-year-old heavy drinker is being investigated for weight loss and obstructive jaundice. An ERCP revealed an irregular lesion distorting the ampulla. Ultrasound and CT scans of the abdomen have revealed an irregular calcified area in the head of the pancreas and extensive calcification throughout the rest of the gland. The radiologist is unable to exclude a malignancy of the head of the pancreas.

88 MANAGEMENT OF CHRONIC PANCREATITIS

1** **E – Enzymatic replacement therapy**
Loss of exocrine function leads to fat malabsorption and steatorrhoea.

2 **C – CT scan of abdomen (with pancreatic protocol)**

- See ERN MRCS Book 2, Chapter 1, section 5.7.

- Of paramount importance is the differentiation of chronic pancreatitis from carcinoma. CT scanning with pancreatic protocol, ultrasound and ERCP provide complementary information.

- The management of chronic pancreatitis is essentially medical, involving: (i) pain management (analgesics/plexus blocks); (ii) exocrine support (orally administered pancreatic enzymes); and (iii) endocrine support (oral hypoglycaemics/parenteral insulin).

89 CARCINOMA OF THE PANCREAS

1** **D – ERCP**

2 **C – CT scan of abdomen (with pancreatic protocol)**
Distal pancreatic lesions are best assessed with CT. Additional information may be obtained at ERCP for head of pancreas tumours.

3 **F – Percutaneous FNAC**
Cytological examination is required to further elucidate the nature of this irregular mass.

- See ERN MRCS Book 2, Chapter 1, section 5.8.

- Imaging techniques to diagnose and stage pancreatic neoplasms include ultrasound, endoscopic ultrasound, CT and magnet resonance imaging (MRI).

- Metastasis, peritoneal deposits, gross posterior fixity and invasion into surrounding structures preclude surgical management.

- Excision is only contemplated when cure is considered possible. Options include pylorus-preserving proximal pancreatoduodenectomy (PPPP) for lesions affecting the head, distal and radical pancreatectomy.

- Obstructive jaundice secondary to head of the pancreas tumours that are unsuitable for resection should be managed by ERCP with stent insertion of a biliary by-pass procedure (life expectancy permitting).

COLORECTAL SURGERY

90   THEME: CHANGE IN BOWEL HABIT

A   Chagas' disease
B   Coeliac disease
C   Colorectal cancer
D   Crohn's disease
E   Diverticulitis
F   Functional incontinence
G   Infective colitis
H   Irritable bowel syndrome
I   Ischaemic colitis
J   Ogilvie's syndrome
K   Pouchitis
L   Rectal evacuatory disorder
M   Slow transit constipation
N   Ulcerative colitis

For each of the following clinical scenarios, select the single most appropriate diagnosis from the above list. The items may be used once, more than once or not at all.

1   A 62-year-old man presents to the surgical clinic with a 7-week history of passing loose stools up to three times per day. Previously, he opened his bowels once daily, passing stool of 'normal' consistency. On direct questioning, he denies the passage of blood per rectum, but reveals a period of constipation preceding the change in stool consistency.

2   A 24-year-old man presents to the surgical clinic with a 12-week history of passing loose non-bloody stools up to eight times per day. Further questioning reveals that he has lost 6 kg in weight over the same time period, and has previously been admitted to hospital for incision and drainage of a perianal abscess.

3   An 82-year-old woman is referred by the orthopaedic SHO with a 1-week history of absolute constipation and gross abdominal distension following repair of a left fractured neck of femur.

4   A 34-year-old woman presents with a 6-month history of intermittently opening her bowels up to seven times per day, passing loose, watery, foul-smelling stool that is difficult to flush away. Routine blood investigations and colonoscopy are normal.

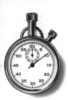

90   CHANGE IN BOWEL HABIT

1   **C – Colorectal cancer**

2   **D – Crohn's disease**

3**   **J – Ogilvie's syndrome**

4**   **B – Coeliac disease**

- See ERN MRCS Book 2, Chapter 1, section 8.

- Colorectal cancer must be considered in a patient of any age presenting with a prolonged change of bowel habit (to looser stools or increased frequency of defaecation) with rectal bleeding and in patients over 60 years with a persistent change in bowel habit only.

- UK Department of Health criteria have been developed to classify those at high risk of colorectal carcinoma warranting urgent investigation (See Thompson MR. ACPGBI Referral guidelines for colorectal cancer. *Colorectal Dis* 2002; 4: 287–297.)

- Colonoscopy is the gold standard investigative procedure, but there is increasing evidence that CT colonography will have an important role in the future.

- Consider functional bowel disorders (which include slow transit constipation, the rectal evacuatory disorders, functional incontinence and irritable bowel syndrome) once organic pathology has been excluded.

91 THEME: BLEEDING PER RECTUM

A   Anal fissure
B   Anal squamous cell carcinoma
C   Angiodysplasia
D   Colorectal cancer
E   Crohn's disease
F   Diverticular disease
G   Internal haemorrhoids
H   Infective colitis
I   Ischaemic colitis
J   Peptic ulceration
K   Radiation-induced proctitis
L   Rectal prolapse
M   Small bowel carcinoid tumour
N   Thrombosed external haemorrhoids
O   Ulcerative colitis

For each of the following clinical scenarios, select the single most appropriate diagnosis from the above list. The items may be used once, more than once or not at all.

1   A 22-year-old man presents to the surgical clinic with a 3-week history of intermittently passing fresh blood per rectum both during and for a short time after straining at defaecation. He does not complain of any pain or the 'feeling of a lump coming down' during the passage of stool.

2   A 70-year-old woman presents to the surgical clinic with a 3-week history of passing fresh blood and mucus per rectum. On further questioning, she denies a change in bowel habit but does reveal weight loss of at least 3 kg over the past month.

3   An 84-year-old man presents to A&E with a 24-hour history of passing fresh blood per rectum unrelated to the passage of stool. He has no associated abdominal pain or change in bowel habit. One year ago he underwent a flexible sigmoidoscopy and barium enema to investigate similar symptoms, although he cannot remember the findings.

   A 67-year-old woman presents to the surgical clinic complaining of regularly bleeding per rectum, associated with a lump that 'comes down' on defaecation that she has to manually replace. Further questioning elicits a long-standing history of constipation, but no recent change in bowel habit. Examination reveals a lump of cylindrical appearance, and no associated external skin tags.

91 BLEEDING PER RECTUM

1   G – Internal haemorrhoids

2   D – Colorectal cancer

3   F – Diverticular disease

4**   L – Rectal prolapse

- See ERN MRCS Book 2, Chapter 1, section 8.1 and Thompson MR. ACPGBI Referral guidelines for colorectal cancer. *Colorectal Dis* 2002; 4: 287–297.

- In any patient presenting with bleeding per rectum and a prolonged change of bowel habit, or those over 60 years with persistent rectal bleeding, the diagnosis of colorectal adenocarcinoma must be considered.

- The colour and nature of the blood passed is often a useful guide to the level of bleeding within the gastrointestinal tract, eg left side: bright red blood; right side: darker and plum-coloured; stomach/small bowel: black, tarry appearance and odour of melaena.

- Bleeding per rectum usually resolves spontaneously with conservative treatment, and can therefore be investigated by endoscopy as an outpatient.

- In the event of refractory bleeding or life-threatening haemorrhage, an attempt should be made to identify the site of the bleed by either endoscopy or angiography. Haemostatic strategies include endoscopic techniques, angiography-guided embolisation and surgery.

92 THEME: INVESTIGATION OF COLOPROCTOLOGICAL DISORDERS

A   Abdominal radiograph
B   Anorectal manometry
C   Barium enema
D   Colonic transit study
E   Colonoscopy
F   Contrast-enhanced computed tomography
G   Endoanal ultrasound
H   Examination under anaesthesia (EUA)
I   Flexible sigmoidoscopy
J   Laparoscopy
K   Laparotomy
L   Mesenteric angiography
M   MRI
N   Proctography
O   Proctoscopy
P   Water-soluble contrast enema

For each of the following clinical scenarios, select the single most appropriate investigation from the above list. The items may be used once, more than once or not at all.

1   A 77-year-old woman presents to the surgical clinic with a 12-week history of passing loose stools up to four times per day. Previously, she opened her bowels once daily, passing stool of 'normal' consistency. On direct questioning she claims she has lost 4 kg in weight. Examination is unremarkable.

2   A 59-year-old man presents to A&E with a 4-day history of colicky lower abdominal pain, increasing abdominal distension and claims he has not passed faeces or flatus for the past 2 days. Examination reveals the patient to have tachypnoea, tachycardia and a rigid, tender lower abdomen. An erect chest radiograph reveals air under the right hemidiaphragm.

3   A 62-year-old man presents to the surgical clinic with an 8-week history of passing blood and mucus per rectum. On digital rectal examination, a mass is noted at 5 cm from the anal verge. Biopsies are taken, and your consultant requests imaging to assess the patient's suitability for surgery.

4   A 45-year-old man presents to the surgical clinic with an 18-month history of recurrent episodes of peri-anal abscesses requiring hospital admissions for incision and drainage. On examination, there are two external openings of fistulous tracts apparent in the 5 o'clock and 8 o'clock positions. Proctoscopy, however, only reveals one internal opening in the posterior midline above the dentate line.

92 INVESTIGATION OF COLOPROCTOLOGICAL DISORDERS

1   **E – Colonoscopy**

2   **K – Laparotomy**
      No imaging is required in unwell patients with peritonitis.

3   **M – MRI**

4**   **M – MRI**

- See ERN MRCS Book 2, Chapter 1, section 8.3.

- Colonoscopy is the investigation of choice in patients with suspected colorectal cancer.

- All patients with rectal carcinoma should undergo preoperative MRI for tumour and nodal staging (TNM classification). MRI assesses the circumferential margin, provides evidence of lymphovascular invasion and helps decide whether neoadjuvant preoperative chemo-radiotherapy is indicated.

- Patients with acute intestinal obstruction but no evidence of perforation should be investigated pre-operatively by either water-soluble contrast enema or a contrast enhanced CT (with or without rectal contrast) to distinguish between mechanical and pseudo-obstruction.

- MRI is the gold standard investigative procedure for evaluation of complicated perianal fistulae, allowing classification of the fistula in relation to the surrounding sphincter complex, and identification of secondary tracts or abscesses.

- Functional disorders of the bowel tend to be assessed using anorectal physiological investigations, which includes anorectal manometry, endoanal ultrasound, colonic transit studies and evacuation proctography.

93   THEME: MANAGEMENT OF COLORECTAL CANCER

A   Abdominoperineal resection
B   Adjuvant chemoradiotherapy
C   Adjuvant chemotherapy
D   Adjuvant radiotherapy
E   Anterior resection
F   Extended right hemicolectomy
G   Left hemicolectomy
H   Neoadjuvant chemoradiotherapy
I   Polyp excision and surveillance
J   Right hemicolectomy
K   Sigmoid colectomy
L   Transanal resection

For each of the following clinical scenarios, select the single most appropriate therapeutic option from the above list. The items may be used once, more than once or not at all.

1   A 62-year-old woman is referred to the surgical clinic with a microcytic anaemia. Examination reveals pallor but no abdominal signs or abnormalities on rigid sigmoidoscopy. Subsequent colonoscopy reveals an irregular lesion within the proximal transverse colon, which proves to be an invasive adenocarcinoma on biopsy.

2   A 54-year-old man presents to the surgical clinic with a 9-week history of the painless passage of fresh red blood on a daily basis. Digital rectal examination and rigid sigmoidoscopy reveal a hard, irregular mass at 6–7 cm from the anal verge. Biopsies indicate a well-differentiated adenocarcinoma, and a pelvic MRI reveals the circumferential resection margins are clear.

3   A 73-year-old woman returns to the surgical clinic following a recent anterior resection for discussion of her histopathological report and the possible need for further treatment. The histological examination confirms Duke's stage C_1 cancer.

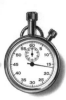

93   MANAGEMENT OF COLORECTAL CANCER

1	F – Extended right hemicolectomy
2	E – Anterior resection
3**	B – Adjuvant chemoradiotherapy

- See ERN MRCS Book 2, Chapter 1, section 8.6.

- Colonoscopy is the gold standard investigative procedure.

- Preoperative screening for lung and liver metastases should be carried out by chest radiography and abdominal CT or ultrasound, respectively.

- Resection is the only advisable primary treatment for proven colorectal adenocarcinoma.

- Chemotherapy and radiotherapy are given either before (neoadjuvant) or after (adjuvant) definitive surgical treatment in attempt to reduce local recurrence and mortality rates.

- The current international adjuvant chemotherapy regimen is 6 months of 5-fluorouracil (5-FU) and folinic acid (FA).

94 THEME: MANAGEMENT OF INFLAMMATORY BOWEL DISEASE

A   Colectomy and ileorectal anastomosis
B   Colectomy with ileostomy and preservation of rectal stump
C   iv hydrocortisone + serial plain abdominal radiographs
D   iv infliximab
E   Limited colonic resection and primary anastomosis
F   Mesalazine (5-ASA) enema only
G   Mesalazine enema + oral mesalazine
H   Oral mesalazine only
I   Oral prednisolone only
J   Panproctocolectomy and permanent ileostomy
K   Prednisolone enema only
L   Prednisolone enema + oral prednisolone
M   Restorative proctocolectomy and ileal reservoir

For each of the following clinical scenarios, select the single, most appropriate therapeutic option from the above list. The items may be used once, more than once or not at all.

1   A 25-year-old man presents to the surgical clinic with a 3-month history of passing loose, bloody stools up to four times per day. Clinical examination is unremarkable, but rigid sigmoidoscopy reveals friable, ulcerated rectal mucosa up to 12 cm, after which the mucosa appears normal in appearance.

2   A 42-year-old woman known to have ulcerative colitis presents to A&E with a 4-day history of bloody diarrhoea up to 10 times per day, associated with severe abdominal pain and distension. On examination, the patient is febrile, tachycardic and palpation of the abdomen reveals non-specific tenderness and distension. Erect chest X-ray is unremarkable, but a supine abdominal film reveals that the transverse colon is 8 cm in diameter.

3   A 30-year-old man is referred to the surgical clinic for consideration of surgery for poorly controlled Crohn's disease affecting the entire colon. Examination reveals multiple anal skin tags and evidence of previous surgery for peri-anal fistulae.

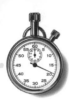

94 MANAGEMENT OF INFLAMMATORY BOWEL DISEASE

1   **G – Mesalazine enema + oral mesalazine**

2   **B – Colectomy with ileostomy and preservation of rectal stump**

3**   **J – Panproctocolectomy and permanent ileostomy**

- See ERN MRCS Book 2, Chapter 1, section 8.4 and Carter MJ, Lobo AJ and Travis SPL. British Society of Gastroenterology guidelines for management of inflammatory bowel disease in adults. *Gut* 2004; 53 (Suppl V): v1–v16.

- Management of ulcerative colitis and Crohn's disease depends on disease activity and location. Activity is graded as mild, moderate or severe according to Harvey–Bradshaw Index and Truelove and Witts' criteria for Crohn's disease and ulcerative colitis, respectively.

- Management of active disease in both ulcerative colitis and Crohn's disease is not dissimilar:

  - Mild to moderate disease – mesalazine (oral and/ or rectal administration), reserve prednisolone, metronidazole, or nutritional therapy (eg elemental or polymeric diet) as second line therapy.
  - Severe disease – iv hydrocortisone, fluid and electrolyte resuscitation, daily examination, serial abdominal X-rays to monitor colonic dilatation.

- Indications for surgery – toxic megacolon (colonic diameter > 5.5 cm or caecal diameter > 9 cm on abdominal X-ray), generalised peritonitis and/or failure of best medical management after 72 hours.

- Emergency operation of choice is colectomy with ileostomy and preservation of rectal stump, with consideration of completion proctectomy on recovery.

- In Crohn's disease, surgery is palliative, not curative.

95 THEME: RIGHT ILIAC FOSSA MASS

A   Actinomycosis
B   Appendix abscess
C   Appendix mass
D   Caecal carcinoma
E   Crohn's disease
F   Diverticular mass
G   Iliac artery aneurysm
H   Iliac lymphadenopathy
I   Inguinal hernia
J   Mucocoele of the gallbladder
K   Ovarian carcinoma
L   Ovarian cyst
M   Pelvic kidney
N   Psoas abscess
O   Spigelian hernia
P   Tuberculous ileitis

For each of the following clinical scenarios, select the single most appropriate diagnosis from the above list. The items may be used once, more than once or not at all.

1   An 18-year-old man presents to A&E with a 4-day history of colicky right iliac fossa pain associated with anorexia and general malaise. On examination, the patient has a temperature of 36.5 °C, a pulse rate 82 bpm and there is a tender, indistinct mass in the right iliac fossa.

2   A 61-year-old man presents to the surgical clinic with anaemia, unexplained weight loss and non-specific lower abdominal pain. On examination there is a hard, non-tender mass in the right iliac fossa.

3   A 57-year-old woman presents to A&E with a 7-day history of colicky right iliac fossa pain associated with constipation and a persistent fever. Direct questioning reveals previous similar episodes of lesser severity. On examination, she has a temperature of 37.8 °C, a pulse rate 98 bpm, an old gridiron scar, and a tender, indistinct mass in the right iliac fossa.

95 RIGHT ILIAC FOSSA MASS

1   C – Appendix mass

2   D – Caecal carcinoma

3**   F – Diverticular mass

- See ERN MRCS Book 2, Chapter 1, section 8.1

- The investigation of choice is contrast-enhanced CT scan of the abdomen and pelvis.

- In the systemically well patient, non-malignant inflammatory masses are best managed conservatively. Follow-up should include repeat contrast-enhanced CT to monitor resolution and consideration of elective resection.

- A swinging pyrexia, persistent tachycardia or generalised sepsis should alert the surgeon to the possibility of an intra-abdominal abscess. Drainage is the best treatment, either under radiological control or surgically.

- Beware the floppy sigmoid colon trespassing in the right iliac fossa, and therefore any associated pathology masquerading as right iliac fossa pathology.

96 THEME: CLINICAL PRESENTATIONS OF DIVERTICULAR DISEASE

A   Acute colonic obstruction
B   Acute diverticulitis
C   Colovaginal fistula
D   Colovesical fistula
E   Diverticular abscess
F   Diverticular mass
G   Diverticulosis
H   Left-sided diverticular bleed
I   Right-sided diverticular bleed
J   Perforated diverticulum

For each of the following clinical scenarios, select the single most appropriate diagnosis from the above list. The items may be used once, more than once or not at all.

1   A 72-year-old woman presents to A&E with a 6-hour history of passing dark red blood per rectum independent of the passage of stool. On examination, her abdomen is soft and non-tender with no palpable masses.

2   A 54-year-old man presents to A&E with a 4-day history of colicky lower abdominal pain, abdominal distension and claims he has not passed faeces for the past two days. On examination, the patient is afebrile and has a pulse rate of 84 bpm. Palpation of the abdomen reveals a firm, non-tender lesion in the left iliac fossa. Digital rectal examination is unremarkable.

3   A 65-year-old woman presents to the surgical clinic with a chronic history of intermittent episodes of lower colicky abdominal pain and general malaise. On direct questioning, she believes her symptoms began 8-months ago after a 2-day period of severe lower abdominal pain which then resolved spontaneously. Further, she incidentally mentions that she often passes air while micturating.

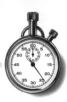

96   CLINICAL PRESENTATIONS OF DIVERTICULAR DISEASE

1   **I – Right-sided diverticular bleed**

2   **F – Diverticular mass**

3**   **D – Colovesical fistula**

- See ERN MRCS Book 2, Chapter 1, section 6.2.

- Diverticular disease most commonly affects the sigmoid colon (95–98%).

- Patients often present with symptoms of lower abdominal pain, distension and change of bowel habit. They should all undergo barium enema, colonoscopy or possibly CT colonography to exclude neoplastic disease. Most will improve by increasing their dietary fibre intake.

- Acute diverticulitis can usually be managed conservatively with analgesia, bowel rest, intravenous fluids and broad-spectrum antibiotics. Failure of symptoms to resolve after 48 hours or the presence of any complicating factors, such as sepsis or palpable masses, should be investigated by contrast-enhanced CT.

- If operation is required, limited resection and primary anastomosis is safe in selected cases.

- There is increasing evidence that elective resection should be offered to patients < 50 years after a single emergency admission, and after two admissions if > 50 years.

97   THEME: CONSTIPATION

A   Anorectal physiology, colonic transit study and evacuation proctography
B   Antegrade continence enema procedure
C   Biofeedback
D   Dietary fibre supplementation
E   Duhamel's procedure
F   Glycerine suppositories
G   Osmotic laxatives (eg lactulose)
H   Manual disimpaction under anaesthesia
I   Phosphate enemas
J   Sacral nerve stimulation
K   Stimulant laxatives (eg senna or bisacodyl)
L   Subtotal colectomy and ileorectal anastomosis

For each of the following clinical scenarios, select the single, most appropriate next step in management from the above list. The items may be used once, more than once or not at all.

☐ 1   A 25-year-old woman presents to the surgical clinic with a 2-year history of opening her bowels approximately once per week, associated with the feeling of incomplete evacuation. Abdominal and digital rectal examinations are unremarkable.

☐ 2   A 34-year-old man returns to the surgical clinic frustrated that, despite trying a variety of laxatives and suppositories, his long-standing constipation has not resolved. He would like to be considered for surgical intervention.

☐ 3   A 19-year-old man with a history of chronic constipation since childhood returns to the clinic to receive the results of a recent rectal biopsy. The histological report states that there are an absence of ganglion cells in the myenteric and submucosal plexus of the rectum.

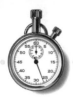

97 CONSTIPATION

1 **A – Anorectal physiology, colonic transit study and evacuation proctography**

2 **C – Biofeedback**

3** **E – Duhamel's procedure**
Involves excision of the dilated rectum and oversewing of the distal rectal stump via an abdominal approach, followed by creation of an end-to-side anastomosis of the proximal bowel to the posterior aspect of the rectal stump via a perineal approach.

• See ERN MRCS Book 2, Chapter 1, section 8.1.

• Constipation is usually 'simple' in nature due to low fluid/fibre intake. It may occur secondary to organic disease of the gastrointestinal tract (eg mechanical obstruction) or extragastrointestinal (endocrine/metabolic/neurological) disorders.

• In the absence of organic pathology, it is termed functional constipation and occurs due to delayed progression of intestinal contents (slow transit constipation) and/or impaired rectal evacuation (rectal evacuatory disorder/outlet obstruction).

• Traditional 'step-up' treatment of simple/functional constipation is:
  – Dietary fibre supplementation.
  – Trial of laxatives, suppositories, enemas and pro-kinetics.
  – Biofeedback (gut-directed behavioural therapy), which appears effective in up to 60% of unselected patients with constipation in tertiary referral centres.
  – Surgery in only very selected cases following comprehensive physiological and psychological evaluation.

• Patients with chronic constipation who fail first-line treatment may undergo anorectal physiological investigations, colonic transit studies and evacuation proctography to distinguish those patients with slow transit constipation and rectal evacuatory disorders to guide further treatment.

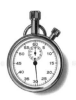

98 THEME: FAECAL INCONTINENCE

A   Anal plug
B   Anorectal physiology, endoanal ultrasound, evacuation proctography
C   Anterior sphincter repair
D   Artificial sphincter
E   Biofeedback
F   Bulking agents
G   Electrically stimulated gracilis neosphincter
H   Glycerine suppositories/phosphate enemas
I   Loperamide
J   Sacral nerve stimulation
K   Stoma formation

For each of the following scenarios described below, select the single most appropriate management option from the above list. The items may be used once, more than once or not at all.

1   A 34-year-old woman presents to the surgical clinic with a 6-month history of urge faecal incontinence following the birth of her first child.

2   A 72-year-old man presents to the surgical clinic with a 1-month history of passive faecal leakage. Examination reveals a mildly distended lower abdomen and a soft indentable mass in the left iliac fossa.

3   A 54-year-old woman with a 5-year history of worsening urge faecal incontinence returns to the surgical clinic, having failed a trial of medical therapy, pelvic floor retraining and behavioural therapy. Investigations to date reveal an isolated deficit in the external anal sphincter and normal pudendal nerve function.

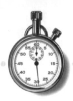

98   FAECAL INCONTINENCE

1   B – Anorectal physiology, endoanal ultrasound, evacuation proctography

2   H – Glycerine suppositories/phosphate enemas

3**   C – Anterior sphincter repair

- See ERN MRCS Book 2, Chapter 1, section 9.10.

- The commonest cause of faecal incontinence in women is obstetric trauma.

- Following a detailed history and careful examination the majority of patients may benefit from conservative medical therapy with anti-diarrhoeals (eg loperamide).

- Anorectal physiology, endoanal ultrasound and evacuation proctography can be used to guide medical therapy or further management in the event of its failure.

- A traditional step-wise approach for the treatment of incontinence in those whom medical therapy has been ineffective is:

    - pelvic floor retraining and biofeedback (gut-directed behavioural therapy)
    - sacral nerve stimulation
    - consideration of direct sphincter repair or sphincter augmentation
    - stoma formation.

- The majority of patients with an identified anal sphincter defect on endoanal ultrasound will benefit from anterior sphincter repair in the short-term. However, only 40% will remain continent in the long term.

99 THEME: ANAL AND PERIANAL PAIN

A	Anal carcinoma
B	Anal chancre
C	Anal fissure
D	Condylomata acuminata
E	Internal haemorrhoids
F	Perianal sepsis
G	Pilonidal abscess
H	Proctalgia fugax
I	Rectal prolapse
J	Solitary rectal ulcer syndrome
K	Thrombosed external haemorrhoids
L	Ulcerative perianal herpes simplex

For each of the following clinical scenarios, select the single most appropriate diagnosis from the above list. The items may be used once, more than once or not at all.

☐ 1 A 25-year-old man presents to the surgical clinic with a 4-month history of severe pain on defaecation persisting for several minutes afterwards. On further questioning, he also complains of the passage of a small volume of fresh blood and constipation. Examination reveals a prominent skin tag at the anal verge in the 12 o'clock position.

☐ 2 A 32-year-old man presents to the surgical clinic with severe perianal pain associated with discharge for the past 3 weeks. Direct questioning reveals a history of regular unprotected anal intercourse. Examination reveals two circular indurated tender lesions opposite each other at the anal verge.

☐ 3 A 45-year-old woman presents to the surgical clinic with an 8-month history of intermittent perianal pain and swelling followed by a spontaneous discharge. Examination reveals a small opening 3 cm from the anal verge in the 2 o'clock position.

☐ 4 An 18-year-old man presents to A&E complaining of severe perianal pain. On examination there is an exquisitely tender, indurated swelling within the natal cleft.

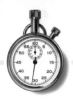

99   ANAL AND PERIANAL PAIN

1   C – Anal fissure

2**   B – Anal chancre

3   F – Perianal sepsis

4   G – Pilonidal abscess

- See ERN MRCS Book 2, Chapter 1, section 9.

- The most common benign anorectal conditions are:

    - Anal fissure: pain on defecation that persists for a few minutes to hours afterwards, often associated with the passage of a small volume of bright red blood.
    - Perianal sepsis: recurrent episodes of perianal pain and swelling followed by spontaneous discharge or need for repeated hospital admissions for incision and drainage of abscesses.
    - Pilonidal sepsis: recurrent abscesses within the natal cleft. They have no relation to the anorectum.
    - Haemorrhoids: uncomplicated haemorrhoidal disease is usually painless. The majority of patients complain of the passage of bright red blood and/ or prolapse. However, thrombosed haemorrhoids are exquisitely tender and there is a clinically obvious blood clot surrounded by oedematous tissue.

- There has been an explosive growth in the prevalence of sexually transmitted diseases of the anorectum over the past 20 years. Recognition of the more common varieties is important, as many produce lesions in the perineum, anus and rectum.

100 THEME: ANORECTAL PROLAPSE

A	Fibroepithelial anal polyp
B	First degree haemorrhoids
C	Fourth degree haemorrhoids
D	Full thickness rectal prolapse
E	Intussusception
F	Mucosal rectal prolapse
G	Second degree haemorrhoids
H	Third degree haemorrhoids
I	Thrombosed external haemorrhoids

For each of the following scenarios described below, select the most appropriate diagnosis from the above list. The items may be used once, more than once or not at all.

☐ 1 A 22-year-old man presents to the surgical clinic with a 3-month history of a lump that prolapses and bleeds on defaecation, which he has to digitally reduce. Examination reveals perianal appendages around the anus, and proctoscopy reveals two friable swellings above the dentate line, which prolapse on straining.

☐ 2 A 51-year-old woman presents to the surgical clinic with a 4-month history of a lump that prolapses and bleeds on defaecation, which spontaneously reduces. Examination reveals no perianal appendages, but proctoscopy and straining reveal a cylindrical muscular tube.

100 ANORECTAL PROLAPSE

1   **H – Third degree haemorrhoids**

2**   **D – Full thickness rectal prolapse**

- See ERN MRCS Book 2, Chapter 1, section 9.8.

- The symptoms of prolapsing haemorrhoids and full thickness rectal prolapse are very similar. The clinical appearances are very different with a full thickness prolapse having a circumferential, cylindrical appearance, whereas internal haemorrhoids appear as enlarged vascular cushions commencing at the dentate line, usually in the 3, 7 and 11 o' clock positions.

- Treatment of haemorrhoids:

  - First degree (bleeding but not prolapsing): high-fibre diet/fibre supplements.
  - Second and third degree (prolapse but spontaneously reduce and prolapse needing manual reduction respectively): rubber band ligation, injection sclerotherapy, or haemorrhoidectomy in refractory cases.
  - Fourth degree (irreducible prolapse): haemorrhoidectomy (stapled or excisional).

- Treatment of symptomatic full thickness rectal prolapse requires surgical treatment.

  - Abdominal procedures (eg rectopexy) have lower recurrence rates but higher rates of constipation.
  - Perineal procedures (eg Altemeier's or Delorme's) have higher recurrence rates but lower rates of functional and systemic disturbance.
  - The PROSPER trial (www.prosper.bham.ac.uk) is currently comparing abdominal versus perineal techniques in a multicentre randomised trial.

101 THEME: MANAGEMENT OF COMMON PROCTOLOGICAL CONDITIONS

A   Abdominoperineal excision
B   Anal advancement flap
C   Botulinum toxin injection
D   Chemoirradiation therapy
E   Dietary fibre supplementation
F   Diltiazem 2% ointment
G   Drainage 'loose' seton
H   Fistulotomy
I   Formaldehyde therapy
J   Glyceryl trinitrate 0.4% ointment
K   Haemorrhoidectomy
L   Injection sclerotherapy
M   Lateral internal anal sphincterotomy
N   Mapping excisional biopsy
O   Proctectomy
P   Rubber-band ligation

For each of the following clinical scenarios described below, select the single, most appropriate management option from the above list. The items may be used once, more than once or not at all.

1   A 34-year-old man presents to the surgical clinic with an 8-month history of persistent perianal discharge. Examination reveals a small opening 2 cm from the anal verge, from which induration can be palpated in a radial direction up to the anus. Subsequent EUA reveals a low trans-sphincteric fistula.

2   A 57-year-old woman returns to the surgical clinic after being recommended an 8-week course of 0.2% glyceryl trinitrate ointment for the management of her anal fissure. Unfortunately, she stopped using ointment after the first week as it caused severe headaches, and her symptoms are no better.

3   A 50-year-old man presents to the surgical clinic with a painful, bleeding ulcer at the edge of the anus. Subsequent EUA reveals further ulceration within the anal canal. Biopsies reveal invasive squamous cell carcinoma.

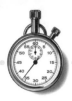

101 MANAGEMENT OF COMMON PROCTOLOGICAL CONDITIONS

1   **H – Fistulotomy**

2   **F – Diltiazem 2% ointment**
More favourable side effect profile than glyceryl trinitrate.

3**   **D – Chemoradiation therapy**

- See ERN MRCS Book 2, Chapter 1, section 9.

- Anal squamous cell cancer:

  - Chemo-radiation is the treatment of choice for most lesions, but consider local excision in small cases at the anal verge. Salvage abdominoperineal excision is reserved for cases that do not respond.

- Idiopathic anal fistulae:

  - Aim of treatment is fistula eradication and sphincter preservation.
  - Surgical fistulotomy ('lay open') ensures eradication but care must be exercised to avoid injury to the (internal) anal sphincter.
  - Setons ('loose' to drain or 'tight' to cut), advancement flaps and fibrin glue are alternative strategies.

- Anal fissures:

  - Chemical sphincterotomy (using diltiazem or glyceryl trinitrate ointment, or injection of botulinum toxin) have good initial results, but high rates of recurrence. Lateral sphincterotomy remains the gold standard of treatment but is associated with an incontinence rate.

BREAST AND ENDOCRINE SURGERY

102 THEME: INVESTIGATION OF BREAST DISORDERS

A   Breast scintigraphy
B   Computed tomography (CT)
C   Core biopsy
D   Ductoscopy
E   FNAC
F   Magnetic resonance imaging
G   Mammography
H   Mammography, ultrasound and FNAC
I   Nipple discharge cytology
J   None
K   Radioisotope occult lesion localisation (ROLL)
L   Ultrasound
M   Ultrasound-guided FNAC
N   Wire-guided excision biopsy

For each of the clinical scenarios described below, select the single most appropriate investigation from the above list. The items may be used once, more than once or not at all.

1   A 67-year-old woman presents to the surgical clinic with an 8-week history of a painless lump in the left breast. Examination confirms the presence of a 1 cm × 1 cm hard, mobile lesion in the upper outer quadrant of the left breast. There are no palpable lymph nodes.

2   A 30-year-old woman presents to the surgical clinic with a 3-month history of pain in both breasts. Direct questioning reveals the pain to be cyclical in nature. On examination, both breasts are non-specifically tender, but there are no discrete lumps palpable.

3   A 27-year-old woman presents to the surgical clinic with a 4-week history of bloody nipple discharge and a lump in the right axilla. Further questions reveals that her sister was recently diagnosed with ovarian cancer. Examination of the right breast and axilla confirms the presence of bloody nipple discharge and lymphadenopathy, respectively. In addition, a P4 lesion in the 12 o'clock position of the right breast.

102 INVESTIGATION OF BREAST DISORDERS

1   H – Mammography, ultrasound and FNAC

2   J – None

3**   M – Ultrasound-guided FNAC

• See ERN MRCS Book 2, Chapter 4, section 1.3.

• All women with suspected breast cancer should undergo triple assessment involving: (i) clinical assessment (P1–5); (ii) imaging – mammography (R1–5) and/or ultrasound (U1–5); and (iii) needle cytology (C1–5) or core biopsy (B1–5).

• Each component of the triple assessment is graded from 1–5: 1 = normal; 2 = benign; 3 = uncertain; 4 = suspicious; 5 = malignant.

• Mammography is the most frequently employed imaging modality. However, it less effective at detecting signs of breast cancer in dense breast tissue (women < 35 years) where ultrasound is the investigation of choice.

• Ultrasound is also used to assess the axilla in women with suspected axillary metastases.

• MRI tends to be used mainly for post-operative disease surveillance, and to investigate women for multifocal disease prior to conservation surgery.

103 THEME: MANAGEMENT OF BREAST INFECTIONS

A   Broad-spectrum antibiotics
B   Broad-spectrum antibiotics + clinical needle aspiration
C   Broad-spectrum antibiotics, clinical needle aspiration + regular expression of breast milk
D   Broad-spectrum antibiotics + regular expression of breast milk
E   Broad-spectrum antibiotics, ultrasound-guided aspiration + regular expression of breast milk
F   Clinical needle aspiration
G   Incision and drainage
H   Ultrasound-guided aspiration
I   Ultrasound-guided aspiration + broad-spectrum antibiotics

For each of the clinical scenarios described below, select the most appropriate next step in management from the above list. The items may be used once, more than once or not at all.

1   A 67-year-old woman presents to the surgical clinic, 1-week post right mastectomy and level II axillary clearance, with a large area of erythematous swelling beneath her mastectomy wound. Examination confirms the presence of fluctuance beneath the wound, with overlying cellulitis.

2   A 19-year-old woman presents to A&E a 4-day history of an increasingly painful mass near the right nipple. Examination reveals a right periareolar tender, fluctuant swelling that is 'pointing' and which measures 3 cm × 4 cm.

3   A 33-year-old woman presents to A&E complaining of a swollen, exquisitely painful left breast. She is breastfeeding her 3-week-old baby. Examination reveals an erythematous, tender, swollen left breast with no obvious focus.

103 MANAGEMENT OF BREAST INFECTIONS

1**   **B – Broad-spectrum antibiotics + clinical needle aspiration**

2   **B – Broad-spectrum antibiotics + clinical needle aspiration**

3   **D – Broad-spectrum antibiotics + regular expression of breast milk**

- See ERN MRCS Book 2, Chapter 4, section 1.7.
- Breast infections can be divided into lactational, non-lactational and post-surgical.
- Lactational mastitis:
  - Occurs in approx. 5% of women who are breast-feeding usually due to *Staphylococcus aureus*.
  - Encouraging regular expression of breast milk and use of broad-spectrum antibiotics reduces the risk of abscess formation.
- Non-lactational mastitis:
  - Two types: periareolar and peripheral.
  - Periareolar mastitis is association with cigarette smoking and usually due to aerobes and anaerobes. Peripheral mastitis is associated with diabetes, steroid therapy and trauma and is usually due to *Staphylococcus aureus*.
  - Rarely, infection is related to underlying malignancy, and a mammogram should be performed in women > 35 years after resolution.
- Post-surgical infection:
  - Usually due to infection of a post-operative seroma.
  - Both chemotherapy and radiotherapy reduce resistance to infection.
- Breast abscesses that are obvious clinically may be aspirated without radiological guidance; all others require (sometimes repeated) assessment and aspiration using ultrasound. Incision and drainage is reserved for abscesses where the overlying skin is non-viable.

104 THEME: GYNAECOMASTIA

A	Biochemical assessment
B	Danazol
C	Drug withdrawal
D	Liposuction
E	Reassurance
F	Surgical excision
G	Tamoxifen
H	Triple assessment

For each of the following scenarios, select the single most appropriate next step in management from the above list. The items may be used once, more than once or not at all.

1 A 14-year-old boy presents to the surgical clinic with a 2-month history of bilateral painful breast swelling. The patient's mother informs you that he experienced similar symptoms in the first few weeks after his birth.

2 A 30-year-old man returns to the surgical clinic with persistent tender left-sided breast enlargement. There are no clear pathological causes, and all appropriate investigations to date have been unremarkable. He declines surgery.

3 A 57-year-old man returns to the surgical clinic with persistent right-sided gynaecomastia despite the recent cessation of spironolactone, which was originally thought to be the causative factor. Examination confirms that his gynaecomastia has not improved; there is non-tender enlargement of the right breast with no associated abdominal or testicular signs.

104 GYNAECOMASTIA

1   **E – Reassurance**

2**   **B – Danazol**
Only medication licensed for treatment in UK.

3   **H – Triple assessment**

- See ERN MRCS Book 2, Chapter 4, section 1.10.
- Triple assessment should be performed if the cause is uncertain or primary breast cancer is suspected.
- Causes can be divided into three groups:

  1. physiological
  2. pathological, including decreased androgen production (eg secondary to renal failure); increased secretion of oestrogens (eg secondary to testicular tumours); increased peripheral aromatisation (eg secondary to liver failure)
  3. drug-induced (eg secondary to steroids, spironolactone, excess alcohol intake, cannabis).

- Treatment:

  - first line: reassurance (physiological); drug withdrawal or replacement (drug-induced); treat underlying cause (pathological)
  - second line: medical therapy – danazol, tamoxifen or clomiphene
  - third line: surgery – options include liposuction and open excision.

105 THEME: MASTALGIA

A	Aberrations of normal development and involution (ANDI)
B	Acute mastitis
C	Breast abscess
D	Breast carcinoma
E	Cyclical mastalgia
F	Fat necrosis
G	Granulomatous mastitis
H	Mondor's disease
I	Tietze's syndrome

For each of the following clinical scenarios, select the most appropriate diagnosis from the above list. The items may be used once, more than once or not at all.

☐ 1 A 24-year-old woman presents to the surgical clinic with a 4-month history of intermittent pain and tenderness within the right breast. On further questioning, the pain is usually worse before her periods and spontaneously resolves shortly afterwards. Examination is unremarkable.

☐ 2 A 31-year-old woman presents to the surgical clinic with a persistent pain deep within the right breast, which is unrelated to her menstrual cycle. On examination, the breasts are normal in appearance and there are no palpable lumps or axillary lymph nodes, however, there is pinpoint tenderness on deep palpation of the upper inner aspect of the right breast.

☐ 3 A 54-year-old woman presents to A&E with a 3-day history of severe pain on the upper aspect of her left breast. On examination, there is erythema over the upper outer quadrant of the left breast, and palpation reveals a thickened exquisitely tender cord-like structure beneath the skin, in the area of concern.

105 MASTALGIA

1   **E – Cyclical mastalgia**

2   **I – Tietze's syndrome**
     A costochondritis that is exacerbated by activity and reproducible on direct pressure to the affected part of the chest wall. Treatment includes rest and non-steroidal anti-inflammatory medication.

3**   **H – Mondor's disease**
     A self-limiting superficial thrombophlebitis of a breast vein. Treatment involves reassurance and non-steroidal inflammatory analgesics.

- See ERN MRCS Book 2, Chapter 4, section 1.4.

- The aim is to exclude sinister pathology and differentiate between true mastalgia (pain within the breast tissue) and referred pain from the chest wall.

- True mastalgia is thought to be of hormonal aetiology and can be cyclical or non-cyclical, although distinction between the two has little clinical importance.

- Mammography should be performed in women > 35 years old, as up to 3% of women presenting with pain are diagnosed with breast cancer.

- Treatment algorithm:

  - First line: reassurance. Advise reduction in fat intake for cyclical mastalgia.
  - Second line: medical therapy – tamoxifen (most effective but unlicensed), danazol (licensed) or bromocriptine (unfavourable side-effect profile).

106 THEME: RISK FACTORS FOR DEVELOPMENT OF BREAST CANCER

A   *BRCA1* gene mutation
B   *BRCA2* gene mutation
C   Early menarche
D   Hormone replacement therapy
E   Late menopause
F   Long-term use of oral contraceptive pill
G   No specific risk factor
H   Nulliparity
I   *TP53* gene mutation

The following patients all have breast cancer. Select the most appropriate risk factor(s) from the above list. The items may be used once, more than once or not at all.

☐ 1   A 67-year-old woman presents to the surgical clinic with a 1-month history of a non-tender lump in her left breast. Triple assessment reveals a P3, U4, C5 lesion. Further questioning reveals she commenced menstruation at 15 years of age. She has had two pregnancies but did not breastfeed with either. Her family history reveals that her maternal uncle was diagnosed with bowel cancer at 78 years.

☐ 2   A 31-year-old woman of Ashkenazi Jewish descent presents to the surgical clinic with a 6-week history of a non-tender lump in the right breast. Triple assessment reveals a P3, U5, B5 lesion. Further questioning reveals she commenced menstruation at 13 years of age, her last menstrual period was 2 weeks ago, and she has never taken the oral contraceptive pill. She has had two children, both of whom she breastfed. Her family history reveals that her mother and maternal aunt were diagnosed with breast cancer at 37 years and 29 years, respectively, and her maternal uncle was diagnosed with bowel cancer at 40 years.

106 RISK FACTORS FOR DEVELOPMENT OF BREAST CANCER

1   **G – No specific risk factor**

2**   **B – *BRCA1* gene mutation**

- See ERN MRCS Book 2, Chapter 4, section 2.4.

- Approximately 5% of breast cancer is hereditary. It is mainly associated with the *BRCA1* and *BRCA2* gene defects, tends to occur in younger women and is often bilateral.

- Certain gene mutations also confer an increased susceptibility to other malignancies, eg:

  - *BRCA1* – ovarian, prostate and bowel cancer
  - *BRCA2* – ovarian, prostate and male breast cancer
  - *TP53* (Li-Fraumeni syndrome) – sarcoma, leukaemia, brain tumour, adrenal cancer.

- Certain ethnic groups have a higher incidence of *BRCA1* and *BRCA2* gene mutations, eg > 2% of the Ashkenazi Jewish population have three mutations (two in *BRCA1* and one in *BRCA2*).

- The remaining 95% of cancers are sporadic, with incidence increasing with age. Risk factors include early menarche, late menopause, nulliparity, long-term use of the contraceptive pill and HRT (all ↑ breast oestrogen exposure).

107 THEME: SURGICAL OPTIONS IN BREAST CANCER

A	Excision biopsy
B	Image-guided guide-wire excision biopsy
C	Image-guided guide-wire wide local excision
D	Image-guided guide-wire wide local excision plus axillary node dissection
E	Mastectomy only
F	Mastectomy plus axillary node clearance
G	Quadrantectomy
H	Wide local excision only
I	Wide local excision plus axillary node sampling
J	Wide local excision plus axillary node clearance

For each of the following clinical scenarios, select the most appropriate surgical option from the above list. The items may be used once, more than once or not at all.

1 A 69-year-old woman underwent a right wide local excision for ductal carcinoma in situ (DCIS) 18 months ago. Despite taking tamoxifen on a daily basis, surveillance mammography reveals two suspicious foci measuring 3 mm and 4 mm in the upper outer and inner lower quadrant respectively. FNAC confirms these to be invasive carcinoma.

2 A 61-year-old woman has a screening detected spiculated lesion in the left breast. Triple assessment confirms an M5, U5, C5 lesion. Histological analysis demonstrates invasive ductal carcinoma.

3 A 57-year-old woman has a screening detected spiculated lesion in the right breast. Triple assessment confirms an M4, U4, B5 lesion. Histological analysis demonstrates DCIS.

107   SURGICAL OPTIONS IN BREAST CANCER

1**   **F – Mastectomy plus axillary node clearance**

2   **D – Image-guided guide-wire wide local excision plus axillary node dissection**

3   **C – Image-guided guide-wire wide local excision**
See ERN MRCS Book 2, Chapter 4, section 2.7.

Breast-conserving surgery
- In single, small (< 3–4 cm) lesions mastectomy and wide local excision have equivalent outcomes in minimising local recurrence and improving survival.

- Breast-conserving surgery produces a more acceptable cosmetic result, and therefore improved body image and lower rates of psychological morbidity.

- Wide local excision should include a 1-cm macroscopic surgical excision margin and the microscopic disease-free margins should be > 1 mm.

- Impalpable screen-detected lesions need to be localised (wire insertion) using ultrasound or mammography (stereotactically guided).

- Wire-guided excision biopsies are performed when fine-needle aspiration and core biopsy have failed to provide a definitive diagnosis.

Management of the axilla
- Axillary node dissection reduces axillary recurrence, but does not improve overall survival. Three levels are described based on the relation to pectoralis minor:

  - Level I – clearance from the lateral border of pectoralis minor
  - Level II – clearance from the medial border of pectoralis minor
  - Level III – clearance from the entire axilla.

- Axillary node dissection complications: seroma formation, wound infection, shoulder stiffness, lymphoedema, damage to motor nerves (especially medial pectoral, long thoracic and thoracodorsal) and numbness of the inner aspect of the arm (intercostobrachial nerve damage).

- Axillary sampling and sentinel node biopsy are used to stage the axilla in those with small, low-grade screen-detected tumours in the hope that the above complications are avoided.

- DCIS has no metastatic potential and does not require axillary dissection.

108 THEME: ADJUVANT THERAPY IN BREAST CANCER

A	Aromatase inhibitors
B	Bisphosphonates
C	Chemoradiotherapy
D	Chemotherapy
E	Chemotherapy, radiotherapy and hormonal therapy
F	None
G	Radiotherapy
H	Radiotherapy and hormonal therapy
I	Tamoxifen
J	Trastuzumab (Herceptin)

The following patients have all had surgery for breast cancer. Select the single most appropriate adjuvant therapy from the above list. The items may be used once, more than once or not at all.

1 A 67-year-old woman recently underwent a left mastectomy and axillary dissection for an invasive ductal carcinoma. Post-operatively, the histology report reveals a 43 mm grade III tumour, ER/PR positive, human epidermal growth factor receptor (HER) 2 negative and two out of seven lymph nodes involved.

2 A 52-year-old woman recently underwent a right guide-wire wide local excision for a 15 mm region of DCIS detected on screening mammography. Post-operatively, the histological report confirms a 15 mm area of high-grade DCIS, which is ER positive/PR negative, HER-2 negative.

DCIS ──→ Image guided wire WLE
Invasive ductal CA ──→ Image guide guid WLE WLA +
                        axillary node disse ஓ

In ucase CA ──→ mastectomy + guidey nod
                  clearance

108 ADJUVANT THERAPY IN BREAST CANCER

1   E – Chemotherapy, radiotherapy and hormonal therapy

2** H – Radiotherapy and hormonal therapy

•   See ERN MRCS Book 2, Chapter 4, section 2.8.

•   Radiotherapy (DXT) after wide local excision confers survival equal to mastectomy, with local control rates of 95% at 5 years, and improved body image.

•   Post-mastectomy chest wall and axillary DXT is offered to women with high risk of local recurrence, which includes those with skin or pectoral involvement as well as the factors covered below.

•   Adjuvant hormonal therapy for premenopausal women with ER positive disease includes tamoxifen and possibly ovarian ablation (surgical or chemical), and in post-menopausal women tamoxifen (a selective oestrogen receptor modulator, which has antagonistic activity in breast cancer tissue) or aromatase inhibitors (eg anastrazole), which reduce oestrogen production.

•   Adjuvant chemotherapy is indicated for patients at intermediate to high risk of recurrence (see St Galen's risk categories). Risk factors include: (i) > 3 positive nodes; (ii) tumour size > 2 cm; (iii) ER negative; (iv) age < 35 years; (v) HER-2 positive; (vi) vascular invasion; and (vii) histological grade 2–3.

•   Two commonly use chemotherapy regimens are cyclophosphamide, methotrexate and 5-fluorouracil (CMF), and doxorubicin and cyclophosphamide (AC).

•   Trastuzumab (Herceptin) is a monoclonal antibody that targets human epidermal growth factor receptor (HER-2), which when over-expressed in breast cancer confers increased risk of local recurrence and worse overall survival. Adjuvant Trastuzumab (Herceptin) has been shown to achieve tumour regression and is considered in patients with HER-2-positive cancers.

109 THEME: EVALUATION OF THYROID SWELLINGS

A   Computed tomography
B   FNAC
C   FNAC and ultrasonography
D   Magnetic resonance imaging
E   Needle core biopsy
F   Needle core biopsy and ultrasonography
G   No investigation required
H   Serum thyroid function tests
I   Thyroid antibodies
J   Thyroid isotope scanning
K   Ultrasonography

From the above list, select the most appropriate method of evaluation for each of the clinical scenarios described below. The items may be used once, more than once or not at all.

1   A 42-year-old woman presents to the outpatient clinic with a 12-week history of a painless swelling in the right side of the neck. There are no other associated symptoms. Examination reveals a 1 × 2 cm lesion to the right of the midline, which moves upwards on swallowing. There are no palpable lymph nodes.

2   A 56-year-old woman returns to clinic following assessment of a clinically apparent thyroid nodule associated with toxic symptoms. Investigations to date reveal a 3 cm right-sided cyst, graded CT2, within a multinodular goitre and suppressed thyroid-stimulating hormone (TSH) levels.

3   An 18-year-old man presents to the surgical clinic with a life-long history of a lump in the middle of his neck, which occasionally gets infected and that he wants removed. Examination reveals a soft, ovoid lump in the middle of neck that moves up on swallowing and protrusion of the tongue.

4   A 29-year-old woman presents to the surgical clinic with a 6-week history of a painless neck swelling. Further questioning reveals recent onset of diarrhoea, irritability and palpitations. On examination, she has upper eyelid retraction, tachycardia and a diffuse midline swelling in the neck with no discrete lesions palpable.

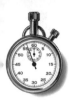

1   **C – FNAC and ultrasonography**

2**   **J – Thyroid isotope scanning**

3   **G – No investigation required**

4   **H – Serum thyroid function tests**

- See ERN MRCS Book 2, Chapter 5, section 1.7.

- Thyroid lesions are assessed using triple assessment – clinical examination, ultrasound and FNAC.

- The main limitation of FNAC is the inability to distinguish between benign and malignant follicular neoplasms. Needle core biopsies, although of high diagnostic accuracy, are painful and more likely to cause complications, such as bleeding, recurrent laryngeal nerve damage and tracheal puncture.

- Measurement of free T_4, T_3 and TSH are used to confirm the diagnosis of hyperthyroidism. Thyroid antibodies (thyroglobulin, thyroid peroxidase and TSH receptor autoantibodies) are found in most patients with Graves' disease and Hashimoto's thyroiditis

- Isotope scanning (eg radioactive ^{123}I or technetium pertechnetate) is most useful in the investigation of a solitary toxic nodule or toxic multinodular goitre, for evaluating metastatic thyroid tumours and localisation of ectopic thyroid tissue.

- CT and MRI are rarely necessary in the initial evaluation of neck lumps but are useful in the staging of malignant lesions.

110 THEME: TREATMENT OF THYROID DISORDERS

A   Carbimazole
B   Carbimazole plus β-blockers
C   Chemoradiotherapy
D   Completion thyroidectomy
E   Hemithyroidectomy
F   Radioactive [131I]
G   Render euthyroid then subtotal thyroidectomy
H   Render euthyroid then total thyroidectomy
I   Sistrunk's procedure
J   Subtotal thyroidectomy
K   Total thyroidectomy

For each of the following clinical scenarios, select the single, most appropriate treatment from the above list. The items may be used once, more than once or not at all.

☐ 1   A 62-year-old woman presents to the outpatient clinic with recent onset of hoarseness, dysphagia and a rapidly enlarging diffuse neck swelling. Cytological assessment reveals giant multinucleated and pleomorphic tumour cells.

☐ 2   A 47-year-old woman returns to the clinic following assessment of a recent thyroid swelling, which she feels presses on her throat when lying down. Investigations indicate a benign multinodular goitre and suppressed TSH levels.

☐ 3   A 53-year-old woman returns to the clinic following assessment of a firm left-sided thyroid swelling. There are no other associated symptoms or signs. Investigations reveal a 1-cm follicular neoplasm.

110 TREATMENT OF THYROID DISORDERS

1** **C – Chemoradiotherapy**
     This is an anaplastic carcinoma.

2   **H – Render euthyroid then total thyroidectomy**

3   **E – Hemithyroidectomy**

- See ERN MRCS Book 2, Chapter 5, sections 1.5–1.13.

- Ensure toxic patients are euthyroid prior to surgery (carbimazole ± β-blockers).

- Solitary thyroid nodule:

    - Toxic: If > 3 cm – hemithyroidectomy; if < 3 cm ablation [^{131}I]
    - Euthyroid: if benign and no pressure symptoms – observe.
    - If benign and pressure symptoms – hemithyroidectomy.
    - If suspicious/malignant – surgery as below.

- Multinodular goitre:

    - Surgery indicated for (5 ms): suspicious/**m**alignant lesions, **m**echanical symptoms (dysphagia etc), failed **m**edical therapy of < ↑ >T$_4$, poor cosmesis (**m**arred beauty) or retrosternal (**m**ediastinal) extension.
    - The current trend is for total rather than subtotal thyroidectomy.

- Papillary and follicular cancer:

    - Papillary cancer (~70–80%) affects young adults and children (paeds); spreads via lymphatics.
    - Follicular cancer (~15–20%); affects older adults (mean fifty years); spreads via bloodstream.
    - Small papillary tumours (< 1 cm) and encapsulated follicular tumours – hemithyroidectomy and TSH suppression.
    - Large papillary tumours (> 1 cm) and invasive follicular tumours – total thyroidectomy and radioiodine ablation (to treat residual disease).
    - Completion thyroidectomy should be performed for follicular tumours with features of invasion following hemithyroidectomy.
    - Thyroglobulin levels are measured post-operatively to detect recurrent disease.
    - Overall, the prognosis is good for these well-differentiated tumours.

- Medullary thyroid cancer:

    - ~8% of thyroid cancers, consider multiple endocrine neoplasia (MEN) syndrome, parafollicular or C-cell origin, spreads via bloodstream and lymphatics, calcitonin is tumour marker.
    - Needs total thyroidectomy and aggressive lymph node clearance.

- Anaplastic carcinoma:

    - Peak incidence 60–70 years, spreads rapidly via local invasion and lymphovascular routes.
    - Surgical resection is rarely possible, and palliative chemoradiotherapy is the main treatment modality.

111 THEME: COMPLICATIONS OF THYROID SURGERY

A	Bilateral complete recurrent laryngeal nerve paralysis
B	Bilateral incomplete recurrent laryngeal nerve paralysis
C	Haemorrhage
D	Hypocalcaemia
E	Hypothyroidism
F	Recurrent hyperthyroidism
G	Superior laryngeal nerve paralysis
H	Thyroid crisis/storm
I	Tracheal collapse
J	Unilateral complete recurrent laryngeal nerve paralysis
K	Unilateral incomplete recurrent laryngeal nerve paralysis

For each of the following clinical scenarios, select the single most likely diagnosis from the above list. The items may be used once, more than once or not at all.

1 A 45-year-old teacher returns to the surgical clinic post total thyroidectomy complaining that on returning to work she has noticed that her voice fades while talking for prolonged periods.

2 A 62-year-old man returns to the surgical clinic 4 weeks post hemithyroidectomy complaining that ever since he was discharged he has difficulty catching his breath while climbing the stairs or on walking his dog. Examination and a subsequent chest X-ray reveal no cardiorespiratory pathology.

3 While on-call the surgical SHO is called to the ward to review a 30-year-old woman 4 hours post hemithyroidectomy. She seems agitated and confused, and examination reveals a pulse rate 140 bpm, respiratory rate 30 breaths/min and a temperature of 39 °C.

111 COMPLICATIONS OF THYROID SURGERY

1   **G – Superior laryngeal nerve paralysis**

2**   **K – Unilateral incomplete recurrent laryngeal nerve paralysis**

3   **H – Thyroid crisis/storm**

- See ERN MRCS Book 2, Chapter 5, section 1.13.

- Recurrent laryngeal damage: unilateral incomplete → slight dyspnoea on exertion/minimal voice change; unilateral complete → hoarse voice; bilateral incomplete → loss of voice/mild dyspnoea; bilateral complete → severe dyspnoea/stridor.

- External branch of superior laryngeal nerve damage → voice weakness/loss of upper half octave in vocal range.

- Parathyroid gland injury → hypocalcaemia. May require lifelong calcium supplements.

- Hypothyroidism – requires lifelong thyroxine replacement

- Haemorrhage is a life-threatening emergency, mainly due to associated subglottic and laryngeal oedema secondary to lymphovascular obstruction. Less commonly, an expanding haematoma can compress the trachea.

112 THEME: DISORDERS OF THE PARATHYROID GLAND

A	Hypoparathyroidism
B	Primary hyperparathyroidism
C	Pseudohypoparathyroidism
D	Pseudopseudohypoparathyroidism
E	Quaternary hyperparathyroidism
F	Secondary hyperparathyroidism
G	Tertiary hyperparathyroidism

For each of the following clinical scenarios described below, select the single, most appropriate diagnosis from the above list. The items may be used once, more than once or not at all.

1 An 18-year-old patient attends the outpatient clinic 4 months following an uncomplicated renal transplant. He is concerned as he is feeling tired and is disappointed that his recovery is taking so long. His plasma calcium is 2.65 mmol/l and serum albumin is 32 g/l.

2 A 24-year-old woman attends A&E 4 days following total thyroidectomy complaining of cramp in both of her wrists and a tingling sensation around her mouth.

3 A 62-year-old woman attends the outpatient clinic with a longstanding history of generalised abdominal pain. There are no other associated symptoms or seemingly relevant past medical history, but the patient incidentally mentions that she is always exceptionally thirsty. Examination is unremarkable. Her corrected plasma calcium is 3.15 mmol/l.

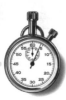

112 DISORDERS OF THE PARATHYROID GLAND

1**   G – Tertiary hyperparathyroidism

2   A – Hypoparathyroidism

3   B – Primary hyperparathyroidism
See ERN MRCS Book 2, Chapter 5, section 2.5.

Primary hyperparathyroidism
- Characterised by ↑ Ca^{2+} and ↑ parathyroid (PTH) levels (↓ phosphate levels in ~50%).

- Causes include single adenomas (87%), four gland hyperplasia (9%), multiple adenomas (3%) and cancer (1%).

- Clinical presentation includes: excessive thirst, fatigue, pathological fractures (bones), renal calculi (stones), abdominal pain (groans) and psychiatric disturbance (psychic moans).

- Bilateral neck exploration cures ~95% of cases, often following pre-operative localisation using **sestamibi scanning.**

Secondary hyperparathyroidism
- Characterised by ↓ Ca^{2+} and ↑ PTH, secondary pathology **extrinsic** to parathyroid gland.

- Most common cause is chronic renal failure.

- Clinical presentation includes bony lesions (eg pepperpot skull), severe itching and metastatic calcification, which can lead to calciphylaxis (mortality ~50%).

- Treatment includes medical therapy (eg Ca^{2+} and vitamin D supplementation) and, if that fails, renal transplant.

Tertiary hyperparathyroidism
- ↑ Ca^{2+} and ↑ PTH secretion, secondary to autonomous parathyroid gland activity, in patients post renal transplant with previous secondary hyperparathyroidism.

Quaternary hyperparathyroidism
- Hypothetical term for tertiary hyperparathyroidism (four gland hyperplasia) that progresses to adenoma formation.

Hypoparathyroidism
- Most common post total thyroidectomy or parathyroidectomy.

- ↓ Ca^{2+} levels leading to perioral paraesthesia, carpopedal spasm and Chvostek's sign (facial muscle twitch secondary to tapping over the facial nerve).

- Treat with calcium supplementation.

113 THEME: DISORDERS OF THE ADRENAL GLAND

A   Addison's disease
B   Adrenal adenocarcinoma
C   Carney's syndrome
D   Congenital adrenal hyperplasia
E   Ectopic adrenocorticotropic hormone (ACTH) secretion
F   Long-term steroid administration
G   Neuroblastoma
H   Phaeochromocytoma
I   Pituitary adenoma
J   Primary hyperaldosteronism
K   Secondary hyperaldosteronism

For each of the clinical scenarios described below, select the single most likely diagnosis from the above list. The items may be used once, more than once or not at all.

☐ 1   A 62-year-old woman attends A&E with abdominal pain, and vomiting; she is convinced that she is going to die. She appears pale and sweaty and her blood pressure is 200/95 mmHg. Abdominal examination reveals no abnormalities. The patient is admitted for observation and appropriate medical management; an overnight urinary collection reveals high levels of metanephrines.

☐ 2   A 54-year-old woman attends the pre-admission clinic in preparation for an elective laparoscopic cholecystectomy. Examination is unremarkable with the exception of a blood pressure of 220/105 mmHg, despite regular anti-hypertensive medication. Serum bloods reveal Na$^+$ 129 mmol/l and K$^+$ 2.3 mmol/l.

☐ 3   A 47-year-old woman is referred to the outpatient clinic for further investigation of Cushing's syndrome. A high-dose dexamethasone suppression test reveals a significant drop in serum cortisol following administration of 2 mg dexamethasone 6 hourly for 2 days.

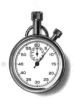

1   H – Phaeochromocytoma

2   J – Primary hyperaldosteronism

3**   I – Pituitary adenoma

See ERN MRCS Book 2, Chapter 5, section 3.

Cushing's syndrome

- ACTH-dependent (↑ cortisol and ↑ ACTH levels) – pituitary adenoma (Cushing's disease) or ectopic ACTH-producing tumours (eg small-cell carcinoma of the lung).

- ACTH-independent (↑ cortisol and ↓ ACTH levels) – adrenal adenoma/carcinoma, adrenal hyperplasia (associated with Carney's syndrome), iatrogenic (eg long-term steroid administration).

- Investigations: 24-hour urinary cortisol and low-dose dexamethasone suppression test (failure of cortisol suppression indicates Cushing's syndrome). Use of CT and MRI to localise and/or characterise lesion (adenoma versus carcinoma).

- Surgery may employ an open approach (suspected malignancy) or laparoscopic (benign tumours) approach.

Phaeochromocytoma (tumour of adrenal medulla)

- Rule of '10's – 10% malignant, 10% bilateral adrenal involvement, 10% ectopic origin (eg neck, thorax, para-aortic, testicular and ovarian).

- Features include refractory hypertension, palpitations and impending doom.

- Investigations: urinary catecholamines and their derivatives; MIGB scan used to localise lesion and metastatic deposits.

- Treatment involves medical control with α-adrenergic antagonists, fluid resuscitation, and where possible laparoscopic adrenalectomy.

Primary aldosteronism

- Excess aldosterone secretion, independent of renin-angiotensin system (↑ aldosterone, ↓ renin levels) → excess resorption of Na⁺ ions, excretion of K⁺ ions and consequently water retention → characteristic presentation of ↑ **blood pressure and ↓ K⁺.**

- Causes include single benign adenoma of adrenal cortex (> 50% of cases – **Conn's syndrome**), nodular hyperplasia of the zona glomerulosa, and aldosterone-secreting carcinomas of the adrenal gland.

- Investigations: aldosterone, cortisol and renin levels. Fludrocortisone suppression testing. CT and MRI scans are useful for localisation of lesions.

- Treatment involves medical optimisation typically employing potassium-sparing diuretics (eg spironolactone) followed by laparoscopic adrenalectomy.

Secondary aldosteronism

- Excess aldosterone secretion due to ↑ renin secretion (↑ aldosterone, ↑ renin levels).

- Causes include renal artery stenosis, nephrotic syndrome, hepatorenal syndrome and cardiac failure.

- Treatment is aimed at underlying aetiology.

continued on p. 204

VASCULAR SURGERY

114 THEME: VASCULAR INVESTIGATIONS

A   Angiogram
B   Ankle-brachial pressure index (ABPI) measurement
C   Arterial duplex scan
D   CT angiography
E   Doppler study
F   Exercise ABPI measurement
G   Magnetic resonance angiography (MRA)
H   Pole test
I   Toe pressure measurement
J   Venogram
K   Venous duplex scan

For each of the following clinical scenarios, select the single most appropriate investigation from the list above. The items may be used once, more than once or not at all.

1   A 31-year-old woman attends the outpatient clinic with recurrent bilateral varicose veins, requesting surgical intervention. She has a past history of deep venous thrombosis.

2   A 45-year-old diabetic man is referred to the outpatient clinic with a history of rest pain and dry gangrene affecting the great toe on the right foot. On examination, pedal pulses are absent bilaterally. ABPI is reduced on the left (0.55) and right (0.45). His creatinine is 225 μmol/l.

3   A 58-year-old man is referred to the outpatient clinic with intermittent claudication affecting his right calf after approximately 0.5 km (50 yards). On examination, the right femoral pulse is present but weak but all other distal pulses are absent. ABPI on the right is 0.7.

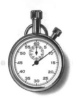

113 DISORDERS OF THE ADRENAL GLAND (cont.)

Addison's disease (adrenal insufficiency)
- Causes include autoimmune adrenalitis (~80%), post-adrenalectomy, hypothalamus–pituitary–corticotrophic dysfunction, cessation of steroids.
- Clinical features include fatigue, anorexia, ↓ weight, hyperpigmentation and ↓ BP.
- Investigations: short Synacthen test.
- Treatment involves steroid therapy.

114 VASCULAR INVESTIGATIONS

1   **K – Venous duplex scan**

2**   **G – MRA**

3   **C – Arterial duplex scan**

- See ERN MRCS Book 1, Chapter 9, section 1.2.

- Do not omit general investigations when assessing vascular patients who have diffuse arterial, and thus multiorgan disease (eg FBC, clotting, U&Es, glucose, lipids, vasculitic screen, ECG, chest X-ray, echo).

- Specific investigations of the arterial system include:

  - ABPI: > 1.1 – calcified vessels; > 0.9 – normal; 0.7–0.9 – mild ischaemia; 0.4–0.7 – moderate ischaemia; < 0.4 – critical ischaemia.
  - When available, arterial duplex is usually undertaken prior to angiography, as it is safer and non-invasive.
  - (Digital subtraction) angiography is usually performed to direct further management once significant disease has been identified on duplex.
  - CT angiography offers a less invasive alternative but does not allow therapeutic intervention.
  - MRA employs paramagnetic contrast substances (eg gadolinium) and is thus safe in patients with renal failure, as the contrast material employed in conventional angiography (and to a lesser extent CT angiography) is nephrotoxic and (relatively) contraindicated in such patients.

- Venous duplex scanning is almost universally undertaken prior to varicose vein surgery and is considered mandatory in the presence of recurrent varicose veins or when concomitant deep venous insufficiency is suspected.

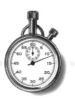

115 THEME: ABDOMINAL AORTIC ANEURYSMS (AAA)

A   Aortogram
B   Assessment of peripheral pulses
C   ABPI measurement
D   CT scan abdomen with intravenous contrast
E   CT scan abdomen without intravenous contrast
F   Duplex scan of arterial system
G   Echocardiogram
H   History and clinical examination
I   Insertion of central line
J   Insertion of two 14G cannulae
K   Insertion of two 18G cannulae
L   Immediate laparotomy
M   Transfer to HDU/ICU
N   Ultrasound scan of abdomen

From the list above, select the single most appropriate next step in the management of the patients in each of the following clinical scenarios. The items may be used once, more than once or not at all.

☐ 1   A 56-year-old man presents to A&E with epigastric pain. On examination he is well, being alert and orientated. His pulse rate is 72 bpm and his blood pressure is 140/94 mmHg. There is an expansile mass present in the epigastrium and all peripheral pulses are present. His haemoglobin concentration is 147 g/l (14.7 g/dl) and his creatinine is 125 μmol/l.

☐ 2   A 50-year-old man is referred by the urologists as he was noted to have a 5.6-cm abdominal aortic aneurysm on an ultrasound KUB to investigate lower urinary tract symptoms. His creatinine is 104 μmol/l.

☐ 3   A 69-year-old woman is brought into A&E following an episode of collapse at home. Her daughter informs you that she has been complaining of abdominal pain that morning. On examination, she is pale and drowsy. Her pulse rate is 120 bpm and her blood pressure is 85/50 mmHg. Her abdomen is distended and both femoral pulses are absent. She has appropriate peripheral access and intravenous fluid resuscitation has been commenced. Her haemoglobin concentration is 83 g/l (8.3 g/dl) and her creatinine is 145 μmol/l.

☐ 4   A 65-year-old man is referred to outpatients with an asymptomatic 5.9 cm infrarenal aneurysm on CT scan of the abdomen.

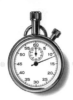

115 ABDOMINAL AORTIC ANEURYSMS

1   **D – CT scan abdomen with intravenous contrast**
Patient has normal haemodynamic parameters.

2   **D – CT scan abdomen with intravenous contrast**
To provide additional information about the morphology of the aneurysm.

3   **L – Immediate laparotomy**
Hypotension in association with abdominal pain/expansile mass suggests a diagnosis of leaking abdominal aortic aneurysm (AAA). The patient is unstable with haemorrhagic shock and thus CT scan is inappropriate

4**   **G – Echocardiogram**
AAA meets criteria for repair. In the elective situation, left ventricular function should be assessed prior to surgery.

•   See ERN MRCS Book 1, Chapter 9, section 2.3.

•   Electively, an expansile abdominal mass may be initially assessed using ultrasound.

•   AAAs are repaired if: (i) symptomatic (pain/pressure symptoms/distal embolic complications); (ii) rapidly increasing in size (> 1 cm/year); or (iii) asymptomatic and > 5.5 cm in maximum diameter, as risk of rupture (> 50% mortality with repair) outweighs risk of elective repair (8% mortality) (UK Small Aneurysm Trial).

•   Repair may be open or endovascular (EVAR).

•   As an AAA approaches 5.5 cm, CT with iv contrast allows more detailed assessment to determine the relationship to the renal arteries (supra/infrarenal) and its morphology to determine whether it is suitable for EVAR.

•   Acutely, investigation is only permissible if the patient has completely normal haemodynamic parameters.

•   Unstable patients need immediate transfer to theatre for laparotomy and repair.

116 THEME: CAROTID ARTERY DISEASE

A   24-hour Holter monitoring
B   Carotid endarterectomy
C   Conservative management
D   CT scan of head
E   Duplex scan of carotid arteries
F   Echocardiogram
G   Medical treatment (anti-platelet/cholesterol lowering medication/β-blocker)

From the list above, select the single most appropriate next step in the management of the patients in each of the following clinical scenarios. The items may be used once, more than once or not at all.

☐ 1   A 75-year-old man presents with a history of collapse. On direct questioning, there is no evidence of transient ischaemic attacks (TIAs) or amaurosis fugax. He has a past history of carotid artery bypass graft (CABG), hypertension and hyperlipidaemia, for which he is currently on medication. A duplex scan reveals a 50–60% stenosis in the right internal carotid artery.

☐ 2   A 68-year-old man presents with recurrent left-sided transient ischaemic attacks. He has a history of hypertension and is an ex-smoker. On examination he is in sinus rhythm. A duplex scan reveals a 70–80% stenosis in the right internal carotid artery.

117 THEME: CAUSES OF LEG ULCERS

A   Arterial   E   Neuropathic
B   Infective   F   Traumatic
C   Malnutrition   G   Vasculitic
D   Neoplastic   H   Venous

From the list above, select the single most likely cause of the ulcers described in each of the following clinical scenarios. The items may be used once, more than once or not at all.

☐ 1   A 42-year-old woman with type 2 diabetes mellitus is referred to the clinic with a chronic non-healing ulcer. On examination, there is an ulcer on the sole of the right foot. Pedal pulses are present.

☐ 2   A 19-year-old woman attends A&E with a painful ulcer on the tip of her right index finger. She describes a history of painful discoloration of her hands during the cold weather. Recently, she has become unwell with general malaise and arthralgia. On examination, she has a facial rash. She is in sinus rhythm and all peripheral pulses are present. Her blood results reveal a normocytic anaemia and an elevated erythrocyte sedimentation rate (ESR).

☐ 3   A 61-year-old man is reviewed in the outpatient clinic. He has multiple ulcers around the gaiter area of both legs. He has a past history of bilateral deep venous thrombosis.

116 CAROTID ARTERY DISEASE

1** **A – 24-hour Holter monitoring**

2 **B – Carotid endarterectomy**

- See ERN MRCS Book 1, Chapter 9 section 4.3.

- Consequences directly attributable to internal carotid artery stenosis include cerebrovascular accidents (CVAs), TIAs and amaurosis fugax.

- Symptoms such as collapse, dizziness etc may represent other cardiovascular or cerebrovascular disease (eg dysrhythmias/vertebrobasilar insufficiency). Formal cardiological investigation and/or neurological evaluation should be performed before consideration for endarterectomy.

- Carotid endarterectomy should be offered to patients with symptomatic (CVA, TIA, amaurosis fugax) stenosis > 70%, as subsequent risk of CVA is 20–30%.

- Debate continues about asymptomatic stenosis > 70% with reduced CVA rates following endarterectomy compared to expectant management in some tertiary centres.

117 CAUSES OF LEG ULCERS

1 **E – Neuropathic**
More likely to predominate in absence of macrovascular disease.

2** **G – Vasculitic**
Patient has systemic lupus erythematosus.

3 **H – Venous**
Secondary to *deep* venous insufficiency.

- See ERN MRCS Book 1, Chapter 9, section 6.4.

- In the presence of peripheral occlusive arterial disease, the 10 times increase in blood flow to allow ulcer healing is not possible. It is associated with ulceration over the pressure areas.

- Venous ulceration characteristically affects the gaiter region and occurs due to chronic venous hypertension, which in turn may be due to superficial (saphenofemoral/saphenopopliteal incompetence) or deep (primary/post-thrombotic) venous insufficiency.

- Diabetic patients are prone to neuropathic (soles of feet) and arterial (macrovascular/microvascular) ulceration.

- Connective disease diseases are associated with Raynaud's syndrome and a generalised vasculitis.

118 THEME: MANAGEMENT OF LEG ULCERS

A	ABPI measurement
B	Amputation
C	Compression bandage therapy
D	Doppler study
E	Duplex scan (arterial and venous)
F	Ligation of saphenofemoral junction
G	Podiatrist referral
H	Revascularisation
I	Skin graft
J	Surgical debridement
K	Thromboembolic disease prevention (TED) stockings

From the list above, select the single most appropriate next step in the management of the patients in each of the following clinical scenarios. The items may be used once, more than once or not at all.

☐ 1 A 75-year-old woman with non-healing ulcers is being managed by the district nurse in the community. She has extensive co-morbidity and requires home oxygen therapy. A previous duplex scan reveals deep venous insufficiency. All lower limb pulses are present and her ABPI is 0.99.

☐ 2 A 45-year-old man is reviewed in the outpatient clinic following a lower limb duplex study, which has revealed bilateral superficial venous insufficiency with saphenofemoral junction incompetence. His lower leg ulcer remains unhealed.

☐ 3 An 83-year-old woman is brought into A&E with painful lower legs and sepsis. On examination, there are several large ulcers affecting the gaiter area, which are malodorous. The base of the deepest ulcer is obscured by slough and extensive black tissue. There is no granulation tissue evident.

☐ 4 A 64-year-old smoker presents with a non-healing right heel ulcer. He has a history of intermittent claudication. On examination, the base of the ulcer is clean. All pulses below the femoral are absent and his ABPI is 0.4. A previous duplex scan revealed a 75–90% narrowing of the superficial femoral artery.

118 MANAGEMENT OF LEG ULCERS

1   C – Compression bandage therapy
2** F – Ligation of saphenofemoral junction
3   J – Surgical debridement
4   H – Revascularisation

- See ERN MRCS Book 1, Chapter 9, section 6.4.
- Principles of wound management dictate that infected, necrotic wounds must first be debrided to allow healing to take place.
- Long-standing/suspicious ulcers require biopsy to exclude malignant change.
- Treatment is directed at underlying cause:
    - Arterial supply must be restored if ulcers due peripheral occlusive arterial disease are to heal. This may require angioplasty or bypass grafting.
    - Deep venous insufficiency – compression therapy (three to four layer bandages), providing that the arterial inflow will not be compromised (ie ABPI > 0.8).
    - Superficial venous insufficiency – saphenofemoral or sapheno-popliteal junction ligation will often promote ulcer healing when secondary to saphenofemoral or saphenopopliteal incompetence, respectively.
    - Diabetic patients should exercise meticulous foot care, visit a podiatrist on a regular basis and seek prompt treatment of traumatic lesions/infection/ulceration.

119 THEME: LEG PAIN

A	Acute cellulitis
B	Acute ischaemia
C	Chronic ischaemia
D	Deep venous insufficiency
E	Deep venous thrombosis
F	Osteoarthritis
G	Ruptured Baker's cyst
H	Sciatica
I	Superficial venous insufficiency

From the list above, select the single most appropriate diagnosis in each of the following clinical scenarios. The items may be used once, more than once or not at all.

1   A 55-year-old man presents with a history of pain in the lower leg. The pain is intermittent in nature and is centered mainly in the calf. It is worse precipitated by walking and relieved by rest.

2   A 35-year-old teacher complains of pains in both legs. The pain tends to affect the medial aspect of both legs and is worse at the end of the day, when she notices some ankle oedema. Clinical examination reveals bilateral varicosities.

3   A 69-year-old man complains of lower leg pain. The pain tends to affect the whole of the outside of the leg down to the ankle. It is present most of the time but gets worse on occasions and is relieved by rest. 'Straight leg raising' is only possible to 45° on the affected side and the ankle reflex is absent.

4   An 82-year-old woman presents with a history of bilateral leg pain. The pain is worse towards the end of the day and is not specifically related to exercise. The pain is relieved by simple analgesics. Clinical examination reveals bilateral restricted knee flexion and crepitus.

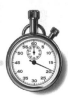

1   **C – Chronic ischaemia**
Defining features of claudication due to chronic peripheral occlusive arterial disease.

2**   **I – Superficial venous insufficiency**

3   **H – Sciatica**
In this case features of lumbar nerve root compression.

4   **F – Osteoarthritis**

•   See ERN MRCS Book 1, Chapter 9, section 3.4.

•   Claudication is feature of chronic peripheral occlusive arterial disease. Criteria for diagnosis are based on the identification of the following specific features: (i) induced by exercise; (ii) occurs after a predictable distance; (iii) relieved by rest; and (iv) experienced in the muscles.

•   It may be difficult to distinguish claudication from osteoarthritis and spinal stenosis as the pain tends to be related to exercise and relived by rest in each. The site of pain (muscles versus joints) and whether the resolution with rest requires the sitting position to be adopted (which implies spinal stenosis) is useful.

•   Aching/pain is commonly associated with varicosities/superficial venous incompetence. It is worse towards the end of the day due to venous hypertension.

120 THEME: LIMB ISCHAEMIA

A   ABPI measurement
B   Amputation
C   Doppler study
D   Embolectomy
E   Routine angiogram
F   Urgent angiogram

From the list above, select the single most appropriate next step in the management of the patients in each of the following clinical scenarios. The items may be used once, more than once or not at all.

1   You are called to see a 74-year-old woman on the orthopaedic ward. She underwent a left hemiarthroplasty 6 days ago and has reported a sudden onset of a painful left leg, which she is unable to move. She denies any symptoms of intermittent claudication in the past. On examination, her right leg is pale and cold. There is no venous engorgement. Her right femoral pulse is present and irregular. There are no distal pulses palpable.

2   A 55-year-old heavy smoker presents to A&E with a 2-day history of worsening lower left leg pain. He previously had a claudication distance of 50 metres and a history of hypertension and hypercholesterolaemia. On examination, the lower leg is dusky and becomes colder towards the foot. The left femoral pulse is present but all distal pulses are absent. His ABPI on the left is 0.5.

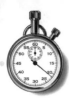

120 LIMB ISCHAEMIA

1   **D – Embolectomy**
Five of the six Ps, which are the hallmark of acute limb ischaemia, are described.

2   **F – Urgent angiogram**
There is evidence of chronic peripheral arterial occlusion.

- See ERN MRCS Book 1, Chapter 9, sections 3.3 and 3.4.

Acute ischaemia
- Characterised by the six Ps: pain, pallor, paraesthesia, perishing with cold, paralysis, pulseless.

- Usually due to distal occlusion by an embolus, although trauma and dissection are alternative causes.

- Treatment options are either: (i) thrombolysis; or (ii) surgical embolectomy. Beware reperfusion injury/compartment syndrome.

Acute on chronic ischaemia
- Previous history of peripheral occlusive arterial disease (claudication etc).

- Acute symptoms suggest either progression of, or thrombus formation at the stenosis, leading to critical ischaemia.

- Urgent angiography is required to further evaluate the stenosis.

121 THEME: MANAGEMENT OF PERIPHERAL VASCULAR DISEASE

A   Above knee amputation
B   ABPI measurement
C   Angiogram – diagnostic only
D   Angioplasty
E   Arterial duplex scan
F   Below-knee amputation
G   CT angiogram
H   Hand-held Doppler study
I   Non-surgical therapy (cessation smoking/exercise/anti-platelet/cholesterol lowering medication (β-blocker)
J   Surgical revascularisation

From the list above, select the single most appropriate next step in the management of the patients in each of the following clinical scenarios. The items may be used once, more than once or not at all.

☐ 1 A 55-year-old man presents with a 6-month history of intermittent claudication. He is currently able to walk approximately half a mile before experiencing symptoms and denies any rest pain or ulceration. He smokes 35 cigarettes per day and is on furosemide for hypertension. An arterial duplex reveals a 70% stenosis in the left superficial femoral artery.

☐ 2 A 67-year-old man attends A&E with dry gangrene of the fourth and fifth toes on his left foot. He has a history of worsening intermittent claudication with recent onset of rest pain. An arterial duplex study has revealed a 70% stenosis in the left superficial femoral artery.

☐ 3 A 73-year-old woman is referred to the outpatient clinic, as she has no peripheral foot pulses. On direct questioning she reports calf claudication after 0.5 km (50 yards) but has recently become confined to a wheelchair following a fractured neck of femur. She has no rest pain or ulceration. On examination, both feet are cool but there are no signs of critical ischaemia. You are able to palpate the femoral and popliteal pulses but no pedal pulses bilaterally.

☐ 4 A 59-year-old smoker is referred with claudication, which has recently evolved to debilitating rest pain in his right calf. On examination the right lower leg and foot is cold and only the right femoral pulse is present. An angiogram reveals multiple stenoses in the superficial femoral artery, which is occluded at the adductor hiatus. The popliteal artery is also completely occluded. The anterior tibial artery reconstitutes via collaterals, providing a single vessel run-off.

121 MANAGEMENT OF PERIPHERAL VASCULAR DISEASE

1 **I – Non-surgical therapy**
   Intervention is based around *clinical* symptoms and *not* radiological findings.

2** **D – Angioplasty**
   Rest pain *is* an indication for intervention.

3 **H – Hand-held Doppler study**
   Her current lack of mobility and absence of critical ischaemia make radiological/surgical intervention inappropriate

4** **J – Surgical revascularisation**
   The occurrence of rest pain demands aggressive intervention. Angioplasty is ineffective in 'small calibre' distal arteries. Femoral–distal grafting is the most appropriate option

- See ERN MRCS Book 1, Chapter 9, section 3.4.

- Chronic peripheral occlusive arterial disease is characterised initially by claudication.

- Critical (as opposed to acute) ischaemia indicates danger to the leg. It may be defined as an ABPI < 0.4 or absolute ankle pressures < 50 mmHg. Practically, it is defined as persistent rest pain or the presence of trophic changes (gangrene/ulceration).

- Arterial duplex/angiography is required to identify the level and degree of occlusion.

- Treatment: (i) exercise/modify risk factors (stop smoking/antiplatelet, antihypertensive, cholesterol-lowering medication); (ii) angioplasty; (iii) bypass grafting; (iv) sympathectomy/vasodilators; or (v) amputation.

122 THEME: VENOUS DISORDERS OF THE LOWER LIMB

A   Anticoagulation therapy
B   Compression stockings
C   Injection sclerotherapy
D   Saphenofemoral junction ligation/long saphenous stripping ± multiple phlebectomies
E   Saphenopopliteal junction ligation ± short saphenous stripping ± multiple phlebectomies
F   Venogram
G   Venous duplex scan

From the list above, select the single most appropriate next step in the management of the patients in each of the following clinical scenarios. The items may be used once, more than once or not at all.

☐ 1 A 45-year-old woman is referred to the outpatient clinic with isolated small varicosities affecting the left calf, which ache and are tender to the touch. Duplex scanning has excluded saphenofemoral or saphenopopliteal incompetence.

☐ 2 A 51-year-old woman attends the outpatient clinic with a non-healing lower leg ulcer. On examination there are varicosities in the distribution of the long saphenous system. Duplex scanning reveals bilateral saphenofemoral junction incompetence and long saphenous reflux.

☐ 3 A 58-year-old man is referred to outpatients with painful swollen lower legs. On examination, there are no obvious varicosities and all peripheral, including pedal, pulses are present. A duplex scan has revealed the presence of deep but *not* superficial venous insufficiency.

122 VENOUS DISORDERS OF THE LOWER LIMB

1**   **C – Injection sclerotherapy**

2   **D – Saphenofemoral junction ligation/long saphenous stripping ± multiple phlebectomies**

3   **B – Compression stockings**
In such a situation, the venous drainage of the lower limb is predominantly via the superficial system of veins given that the deep veins are incompetent. Surgery on the superficial veins will thus interrupt this pathway and is contraindicated. Compression stockings will provide symptomatic relief.

- See ERN MRCS Book 1, Chapter 9, section 6.3.

- Varicose veins may be primary, secondary (to obstruction) or recurrent.

- Symptoms include ache, itch and unacceptable cosmesis.

- Complications include bleeding and chronic venous hypertension (CVH).

- CVH may lead to lipodermatosclerosis and ulceration.

- Established treatment includes:

    – Compression (class II) stockings.
    – Injection sclerotherapy – most effective for small symptomatic veins in the absence of significant venous incompetence.
    – Surgery – 'flush' ligation at the junction with the deep system with stripping (to reduce recurrent rates) remains the gold standard.

- Alternative treatment includes: (i) foam injection; (ii) radiofrequency ablation; or (iii) subfascial endoscopic perforator surgery.

123 THEME: THE SWOLLEN LEG

A	Congestive cardiac failure
B	Deep venous insufficiency
C	Deep venous thrombosis
D	Gravitational oedema
E	Hepatic insufficiency
F	Primary lymphoedema
G	Renal failure
H	Secondary lymphoedema
I	Superficial venous insufficiency

For each of the following clinical scenarios, select the single most likely diagnosis from the list above. The items may be used once, more than once or not at all.

1 A 31-year-old woman attends the outpatient clinic with intermittent ankle swelling, which worse at the end of the day. On examination, there is evidence of varicosities affecting both thighs.

2 A 72-year-old man presents with bilaterally lower leg swelling. Past history includes myocardial infarction. Cardiovascular examination reveals a gallop rhythm. Abdominal examination reveals hepatomegaly. There are no obvious abnormalities of the lower legs other than pitting oedema bilaterally. Serum albumin level is within normal limits.

3 A 68-year-old woman is referred to the vascular clinic with unilateral leg swelling. Past history includes a radical vulvectomy for vulva cancer 12 months ago. Abdominal examination is unremarkable. There is diffuse swelling of the right leg but no other obvious abnormalities.

123 THE SWOLLEN LEG

1   I – Superficial venous insufficiency

2   A – Congestive cardiac failure

3**   H – Secondary lymphoedema
In this case secondary to inguinal lymphadenectomy during radical vulvectomy.

- See ERN MRCS Book 1, Chapter 9, section 6.5.

- Primary lymphoedema may be congenital or idiopathic (Milroy's disease, lymphoedema praecox/tarda).

- Secondary lymphoedema most commonly follows excision of axillary or groin lymph nodes. Other causes include post radiotherapy, malignancy and infiltration.

- Right-sided heart failure leads to peripheral congestion and is a common cause of bilateral leg swelling. By contrast, oedema in hepatic insufficiency is due to hypoalbuminaemia.

ORGAN TRANSPLANTATION

124 THEME: ORGAN DONATION

A Absolute contraindication
B Brainstem death to be tested once again
C Brainstem death to be tested twice again
D No contraindication
E Relative contraindication

From the list above pick the single most appropriate answer for each of the following clinical scenarios. The items may be used once, more than once or not at all.

1 A 45-year-old woman sustains a severe head injury in a road traffic accident and she is certified as having brainstem death. Her family is very keen to donate her organs. She has a history of DCIS of the breast.

2 A 22-year-old man who was previously fit is admitted to the intensive care unit following a subarachnoid haemorrhage. His condition worsens and he is dependent on mechanical life support. The family is keen to donate his organs should such a scenario arise. Brainstem tests were done by the head of the local transplant team and brainstem death is confirmed.

3 A 55-year-old man is admitted in the ICU with intra-abdominal sepsis and septicaemia. He is certified dead. His family inform you that he carries a donor card.

125 THEME: GRAFT TYPES

A Autograft
B Heterotopic allograft
C Orthotopic allograft
D Syngenic graft (Isograft)
E Xenograft

From the list above pick the single most appropriate answer for each of the following clinical scenarios. The items may be used once, more than once or not at all.

1 A 45-year-old man receives a non-related kidney transplant for end-stage renal disease.

2 A 35-year-old woman undergoes a liver transplant for end-stage primary biliary cirrhosis from a non-related donor.

3 A 40-year-old man with Hodgkin's lymphoma had a bone marrow stem cell harvest, which was subsequently given back to him after conditioning chemotherapy.

124 ORGAN DONATION

1   D – No contraindication
2** C – Brainstem death to be tested twice again
3   A – Absolute contraindication

• See ERN MRCS Book 1, Chapter 11, section 9.2.

• The presence of malignancy is an absolute contraindication. Exceptions include carcinoma in-situ, low-grade central nervous system tumours and non-melanoma skin cancer.

• HIV, hepatitis B and active systemic sepsis are also absolute contraindications.

• Tests of brainstem death should be done by two clinicians on two separate occasions and *neither* should be connected with the transplant team.

125 GRAFT TYPES

1   B – Heterotopic allograft
2   C – Orthotopic allograft
3   A – Autograft

• See ERN MRCS Book 1, Chapter 11, section 9.2.

• Autograft – within the same individual.

• Isograft – between genetically identical (syngeneic) recipients, eg monozygotic twins.

• Allograft – genetically non-identical members of the same species.

• Xenograft – between members of different species

• Orthotopic – graft is placed in its usual anatomical location (heart/lung transplant).

• Heterotopic – graft is placed in an abnormal anatomical location (renal).

OTORHINOLARYNGOLOGY, HEAD AND NECK SURGERY

126 THEME: FOREIGN BODIES

A	Clinical examination	D	Examination of oropharynx,
B	Clinical examination and chest X-ray		laryngoscopy, chest X-ray and lateral soft tissue neck
C	Emergency rigid oesophagoscopy	E	No investigation required
		F	Trial of bread, reassure and discharge

From the list above, select the single, most appropriate management for each of the following clinical scenarios. The items may be used once, more than once or not at all.

☐ 1 A 3-year-old boy attends A&E, having been witnessed swallowing a coin. He is pain free and interacting normally.

☐ 2 A 78-year-old woman presents to A&E having choked on a fish bone. She reports that it remains 'stuck behind her jaw bone'. She is now swallowing normally and is comfortable at rest.

☐ 3 A 43-year-old man chokes on a piece of meat and attends A&E reporting that it remains stuck, as he points to his neck at the level of the hyoid bone. Clinical examination and investigation is unremarkable.

127 THEME: INFECTIVE DISORDERS OF THE EAR

A	Emergency myringotomy
B	Elective myringotomy ± grommet placement
C	Hearing test and tympanography
D	Microsuction and topical antibiotics
E	Oral antibiotics
F	Otowick/glycerin and ichthammol wick and discharge
G	Otowick/glycerin and ichthammol wick and review
H	Six-week course of clotrimazole (Canesten) drops

From the list above, select the single most appropriate management option for each of the following clinical scenarios. The items may be used once, more than once or not at all.

☐ 1 A 3-year-old boy presents to outpatients with a history of delayed speech development. Examination reveals a lustreless tympanic membrane with several visible 'bubbles'.

☐ 2 A 29-year-old man post radical cortical mastoidectomy presents with a three-month history of discharge from the ear. Examination reveals a chronic perforation, although his original surgery preserved the tympanic membrane.

☐ 3 A 33-year-old woman presents with several days of tinnitus, jaw pain and headache. Examination is difficult due to an oedematous canal and poor patient compliance.

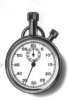

---

1   B – Clinical examination and chest X-ray

2**   D – Examination of oropharynx, laryngoscopy, chest X-ray and lateral soft tissue neck

3   C – Emergency rigid oesophagoscopy

•   See ERN MRCS Book 2, Chapter 3, section 4.2.

•   All patients should have a full history and examination of the mouth, oropharynx and larynx.

•   Radio-opaque foreign bodies (eg coins and bony fish) demonstrated on X-ray to be below the diaphragm may be treated conservatively.

•   Fish bones tend to embed in the valleculae and pyriform fossae, which must be thoroughly examined using direct or indirect laryngoscopy.

•   All patients whose symptoms do not subside must undergo emergency rigid oesophagoscopy as the risk of perforation and mediastinitis is high.

---

127   INFECTIVE DISORDERS OF THE EAR

1   B – Elective myringotomy ± grommet placement
     Diagnosis is chronic otitis media with effusion.

2   D – Microsuction and topical antibiotics
     Diagnosis is chronic infected perforation.

3**   G – Otowick/glycerin and ichthammol wick and review
     Diagnosis is otitis externa.

•   See ERN MRCS Book 2, Chapter 3, section 1.5.

•   Appropriate treatment of otitis media with effusion ('glue ear') is EUA and myringotomy followed by grommet placement if appropriate. Hearing tests would be appropriate prior to surgery in an older child.

•   Oral antibiotics are almost never indicated in otitis externa, although they are in acute otitis media. The risk of sensorineural hearing loss associated with topical antibiotic use in perforation is irrelevant in following previous mastoidectomy, given the profound hearing loss usually associated with this procedure.

•   Otowick or glycerin and ichthammol impregnated gauze is appropriate treatment for a patient with an oedematous canal. Patients must always be reviewed several days later for further treatment and removal of the wick.

---

128 THEME: EPISTAXIS

A Adrenaline-soaked ribbon gauze
B Emergency examination under anaesthesia (EUA) and packing in theatre ±
   submucous resection (SMR)
C Emergency ligation of the external carotid artery
D Local anaesthetic spray and chemical/electrical cautery
E Manual packing and Foley catheter or Brighton balloon
F Manual packing with BIPP pack
G Packing with nasal tampon (Merocel)
H Reassure and discharge
I Refer to ENT outpatient clinic

From the list above, select the single most appropriate next step in management for each of the following clinical scenarios. Assume that appropriate resuscitation has been performed. The items may be used once, more than once or not at all.

1 A 15-year-old boy presents for the fourth time to casualty with minor bleeding from Little's area. Attempts at direct pressure to arrest the bleeding prove unsuccessful. An obvious bleeding point can be easily identified.

2 You are 'fast bleeped' to the resuscitation area of casualty to treat a frail 78-year-old woman with a major epistaxis. She has a background of ischaemic heart disease and, despite nasal packing and adequate resuscitation, is failing to maintain her blood pressure.

3 A 50-year-old woman presents to casualty with a 6-day history of ongoing bleeding from both nostrils. She tells you she has a history of Osler–Weber–Rendu syndrome. Although the casualty SHO has packed the nose with a Merocel (nasal tampon), the patient is continuing to bleed. Examination reveals brisk bleeding from both nostrils and a significantly deviated nasal septum. The patient has a haemoglobin of 73 g/l (7.3 g/dl).

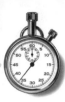

128 EPISTAXIS

1   **D – Local anaesthetic spray and chemical/electrical cautery**

2**   **C – Emergency ligation of external carotid artery**

3**   **B – Emergency EUA and packing in theatre ± SMR**

- See ERN MRCS Book 2, Chapter 3, section 2.4.

- Bleeding from Little's area can be treated with direct pressure, cauterisation or anterior packing of the nose (with either nasal tampons or manual packing).

- Bleeding from an unidentified site requires nasal packing and packing of the postnasal space or use of a 'Brighton balloon'.

- Surgical treatment is indicated in ongoing bleeding with septal deviation or major life threatening haemorrhage.

- Surgical options include SMR in cases of septal deviation, selective vessel embolisation or ligation of ethmoidal or external carotid artery.

129 THEME: NECK LUMPS

A	Branchial cyst	F	Pleomorphic adenoma
B	Cystic hygroma	G	Ranula
C	Lymph node	H	Thyroglossal cyst
D	Mucoepidermoid tumour	I	Thyroid cyst
E	Multinodular goitre		

From the list above, select the single most likely diagnosis for each of the following clinical scenarios. The items may be used once, more than once or not at all.

1 A 23-year-old patient presents to the outpatient department with a 3-month history of a Bell's palsy that was initially treated by the general practitioner with steroids. The patient has been referred to the ear, nose and throat (ENT) outpatient clinic as the palsy has failed to recover. Clinical examination reveals a fullness in the left preauricular area and palpable digastric lymph nodes.

2 A 30-year-old woman presents with a several week history of a midline neck lump. It has become swollen and inflamed. She complains of an odd sensation when she swallows. Examination reveals a fluctuant tender midline mass. It moves upwards on protrusion of the tongue.

3 A 22-year-old man presents with a firm swelling in the upper portion of the anterior triangle of the neck. It is smooth, mobile and non-tender. The patient has been otherwise well. Fine-needle aspiration performed in clinic reveals a yellow–creamy aspirate.

130 THEME: SALIVARY GLAND DISORDERS

A	Calculus	E	Sialoadenitis (bacterial)
B	Cystadenoma lymphomatosum	F	Sjögren's syndrome
C	Mumps	G	Squamous cell carcinoma
D	Pleomorphic adenoma		

From the list above, select the single most appropriate diagnosis for each of the following clinical scenarios. The items may be used once, more than once or not at all.

1 A 78-year-old man presents with a several month history of swelling anterior to the angle of his mandible. Examination reveals bilaterally diffusely enlarged parotid glands with normal facial nerve function.

2 A 22-year-old woman presents with recurrent episodes of parotitis, treated with intravenous antibiotics. On examination, her vital signs are within normal limits and she is apyrexial. Her blood results reveal a white cell count of 6×10^9/l and an ESR of 37 mm/h.

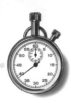

129 NECK LUMPS

1 **D – Mucoepidermoid tumour**
Resulting in invasion of the facial nerve.

2 **H – Thyroglossal cyst**

3** **A – Branchial cyst**

- See ERN MRCS Book 2, Chapter 3, section 6.3.

- 80% of parotid tumours are benign (most commonly pleomorphic adenoma or cystadenoma – Warthin's tumour). Rapid enlargement and involvement of the facial nerve raises suspicion of malignant change. Mucoepidermoid and squamous cell carcinoma are the commonest malignant parotid tumours.

- Thyroglossal cysts are always midline and may present anywhere from the base of the tongue to the thyroid isthmus.

- Branchial cysts present in the third and fourth decade. Commonly sited deep to the superior portion of sternomastoid in the anterior triangle. Aspiration of creamy fluid is diagnostic. Elective excision of the cyst and tract should be undertaken.

130 SALIVARY GLAND DISORDERS

1** **B – Cystadenoma lymphomatosum (Warthin's tumour)**

2 **F – Sjögren's syndrome**

- See ERN MRCS Book 2, Chapter 3, sections 7.4 and 7.5.

- Warthin's tumour, cystadenoma lymphomatosum (also known as adenolymphoma) is a common benign tumour of the parotid. It is bilateral in 10% of cases.

- In all cases of non-resolving parotitis or salivary gland inflammation, Sjögren's syndrome must be suspected, especially in a young female patient with an isolated raised ESR.

131 THEME: HEAD AND NECK MALIGNANCY

A	Excision biopsy of lymph node
B	Excision biopsy of salivary gland
C	Excision biopsy of salivary gland and lymph node
D	Radical neck dissection
E	Superficial parotidectomy
F	Tonsillectomy
G	Total parotidectomy
H	Ultrasound and FNAC
I	Ultrasound, FNAC and panendoscopy
J	Ultrasound, FNAC and tonsillectomy

From the list above, select the single most appropriate next step in management for each of the following clinical scenarios. The items may be used once, more than once or not at all.

◻ 1 A 45-year-old woman presents with a hard fixed swelling under the right side of the mandible. FNAC reveals a squamous cell carcinoma. She attends the pre-admission clinic, reporting a new anterior cervical lymph node.

◻ 2 A 79-year-old smoker presents with a 6-month history of weight loss and several craggy feeling lymph nodes in the right anterior chain. The remainder of the clinical examination is unremarkable.

◻ 3 A 19-year-old girl is referred by the haematologists. She has a several month history of repeated illnesses and her blood film reveals a marked lympho-cytosis and bone marrow suppression. FNAC of a posterior triangle lymph node suggests 'probable lymphoma'.

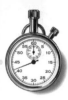

131 HEAD AND NECK MALIGNANCY

1**   H – Ultrasound and FNAC

2   I – Ultrasound, FNAC and panendoscopy

3   A – Excision biopsy of lymph node

- See ERN MRCS Book 2, Chapter 3, section 6.

- 'Individual' metastatic lymph nodes should not be excised. FNAC and ultrasound followed by radical neck dissection is the only acceptable treatment as removal of a single node alters lymphatic drainage in the neck.

- FNAC and ultrasound are the investigations of choice for any suspected malignancy of the head and neck. If there is no obvious primary, then a full ENT examination (known as panendoscopy) should be performed. This includes fibre-optic examination of the nose, sinuses and post-nasal space and direct laryngoscopy under general anaesthetic.

- Excision biopsy of individual lymph nodes can be safely performed in cases of suspected lymphoma.

132 THEME: HOARSENESS

A Functional aphonia
B Globus pharyngitis
C Laryngeal carcinoma
D Recurrent laryngeal nerve palsy
E Reflux oesophagitis
F Reinke's oedema
G Singer's nodules
H Vocal cord papilloma

From the list above, select the single most likely diagnosis for each of the following clinical scenarios. The items may be used once, more than once or not at all.

1 A 19-year-old woman presents with a several month history of something 'stuck in her throat'. She is also experiencing episodes of hoarseness and recurrent chest infections. She has no history of acid brash or retrosternal pain. Examination of the vocal folds is grossly normal.

2 A 56-year-old man with a 6-month history of dysphonia and weight loss is referred by his general practitioner following several episodes of coughing following eating solid foods. Haematological investigations reveal a haemoglobin concentration of 96 g/l (9.6 g/dl).

3 A 56-year-old schoolteacher presents with episodes of dysphonia. She is otherwise fit and well and microlaryngoscopy reveals several small polypoid thickenings on the medial aspect of both vocal folds. The cords look thickened and oedematous.

4 A 60-year-old woman presents with worsening dysphonia. Examination reveals that her left vocal cord is lying in the paramedian position.

132 HOARSENESS

1**   **E – Reflux oesophagitis**

2   **C – Laryngeal carcinoma**

3   **G – Singer's nodules**

4   **D – Recurrent laryngeal nerve palsy**

- See ERN MRCS Book 2, Chapter 3, section 5.3.

- The sensation of a foreign body in the throat is often globus pharyngitis, but in this case when associated with cough and hoarseness is more likely to represent reflux oesophagitis. These atypical symptoms commonly exist **without** typical symptoms of reflux.

- Microcytic anaemia in this age group is most likely to be chronic disease, which in conjunction with dysphonia and dysphagia is likely to represent a malignancy of the larynx.

- Singers nodules are common in 'high demand' voice users such as teachers, singers etc. They do not require investigation and often respond to speech and language therapy.

- Recurrent laryngeal nerve palsy is associated with head and neck surgery, thyroidectomy and apical lung tumours. The left is most commonly affected and the cord lies in the paramedian position due to a failure of adduction.

133 THEME: DISORDERS OF THE TONSILS

A Adenotonsillectomy
B Antibiotics and paracetamol gargle
C Emergency haemostatic surgery
D Local application of adrenaline soaked gauze and hydrogen peroxide gargle
E Needle aspiration
F Six months of combination antibiotic therapy
G Tonsillectomy
H Tonsillectomy and focused radiotherapy

From the list above, select the single most appropriate next step in management for each of the following clinical scenarios. The items may be used once, more than once or not at all.

☐ 1 A 34-year-old woman, who has recently arrived from the Indian subcontinent, presents with a persistent sore throat, fever and night sweats. Examination reveals a unilaterally enlarged tonsil and matted lymph nodes around the neck.

☐ 2 A 14-year-old boy presents with trismus and salivary pooling. It is difficult to examine his throat, but he appears to have a shift of the uvula and a right paratonsillar swelling.

☐ 3 A 9-year-old boy is brought to casualty by his mother with a 15-day history of sore throat and fever. He has some small cervical lymph nodes and bilateral enlargement of the tonsils.

☐ 4 You are fast bleeped to the recovery area of theatres to see a 7-year-old child immediately following tonsillectomy. He has just coughed up a small clot and has blood stained sputum. As the child is very distressed, examination is unrewarding.

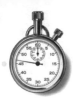

133 DISORDERS OF THE TONSILS

1**   F – Six months of combination antibiotics
       The diagnosis is most likely 'scrofula'.

2   E – Needle aspiration
       The diagnosis is quinsy.

3   B – Antibiotics and paracetamol gargle
       The diagnosis is tonsillitis.

4   C – Emergency haemostatic surgery
       The diagnosis is post-tonsillectomy bleed.

- See ERN MRCS Book 2, Chapter 3, section 4.2.

- Scrofula describes tuberculous infection of cervical lymph nodes and is characterised by unilateral tonsillitis and matted lymph nodes. It is still seen in and arises through drinking milk infected with bovine tuberculosis. Diagnosis is confirmed by excision biopsy of a lymph node and the tonsil. Treatment entails 6 months of combination antibiotics.

- Quinsy refers to a peritonsillar abscess (invariably behind the upper pole). It does not resolve spontaneously and requires needle aspiration, often performed under local anaesthesia. Tonsillectomy is advised 2–3 months later.

- Although 80% of cases are viral, antibiotics are required for persistent infection in tonsillitis.

- Primary post-tonsillectomy bleeding is often due to a loose tie or 'missed vessel'. The treatment is always reoperation, even if the bleeding appears to have ceased. Secondary haemorrhage, if minor, may be managed with adrenaline-soaked gauze and hydrogen peroxide gargles.

134 THEME: EYE TRAUMA

A   Corneal abrasion
B   Lacrimal duct injury
C   No significant injury
D   Orbital cellulitis
E   Orbital fracture
F   Penetrating injury to globe
G   Soft tissue only injury
H   Zygomatic fracture

From the list above, select the single most likely diagnosis in each of the following clinical scenarios. The items may be used once, more than once or not at all.

1   A 16-year-old boy attends casualty after falling from a tree. The only apparent injury is a small laceration to the lower medial edge of his eyelid. Visual acuity is normal and there is no visible damage to the conjunctiva, iris or retina. He wishes to go home.

2   A 40-year-old woman attends A&E following an alleged assault with a broken glass. She has minor cuts to the face, and no visible injury, but there appears to be a small sliver of glass in the left anterior chamber of the eye. She is complaining of ipsilateral blurred vision.

3   A 27-year-old male attends casualty after a night out. He has been drinking and has sustained a blunt injury to his left cheek. He is complaining of double vision. On examination, there is a small subconjunctival haemorrhage.

4   A 17-year-old boy presents to casualty complaining of loss of vision and extreme pain in his left eye following a 'finger injury' during a rugby match. On examination, there is a profuse watery discharge from the affected eye but both eyes feel normal and 'full'. The pupils are equal and reactive bilaterally. The pain settles with the application of topical amethocaine.

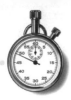

134 EYE TRAUMA

1**   **B – Lacrimal duct injury**

2   **F – Penetrating injury to globe**

3   **E – Orbital fracture**

4   **A – Corneal abrasion**
      Loss of vision is due to perfuse watering.

- Even apparently insignificant lid trauma can cause lacrimal duct damage at the medial lid margin.

- Penetrating eye trauma is an emergency. It is characterised by ↓ visual acuity, visible injury, a 'soft eye' (or ↓ intraocular pressure) and a distorted iris. The presence of an intraocular foreign body is diagnostic.

- Orbit and zygomatic fractures should be suspected where there is evidence of a 'palpable step', diplopia, subconjunctival haemorrhage or significant injury. Facial view X-rays are diagnostic.

- Corneal abrasion may be diagnosed in the presence of a typical history supported by observation of an abrasion following application of fluorescein dye or the abolition of pain following the administration of topical amethocaine (indicates trauma **limited** to the cornea).

135 THEME: OPHTHALMIC INFECTIONS

A   Bacterial conjunctivitis
B   *Candida albicans*
C   Corneal abrasion
D   Cytomegalovirus (CMV) infection
E   Keratitis
F   Ophthalmic herpes
G   Viral conjunctivitis

From the list above, select the single most likely diagnosis for each of the following clinical scenarios. The items may be used once, more than once or not at all.

1   A 39-year-old homosexual male presents to the emergency eye clinic with a unilateral gradual loss of vision. He denies any other pathology, but has a CD4 count of 40 cells/μl. Funduscopy reveals a 'pizza pie' appearance with evidence of retinal haemorrhage, necrosis and retinitis.

2   A 5-year-old boy presents to his GP with a honey-coloured discharge from his left eye. Examination reveals an injected sclera and visible crusting at the lid margins.

3   A 78-year-old woman with advanced metastatic ovarian cancer presents to the emergency eye clinic with severe pain affecting her left eye associated with periorbital tingling. On examination, there is ipsilateral reduced visual acuity and evidence of punctate epithelial keratitis.

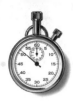

1**   **D – CMV infection**

2   **A – Bacterial conjunctivitis**

3**   **F – Ophthalmic herpes**

- See ERN MRCS Book 2, Chapter 3, section 8.2.

- CMV infection is common in 30% of people with acquired immune deficiency syndrome (AIDS) and is one of the defining illnesses of the disease.

- Ophthalmic herpes reflects reactivation of the herpes zoster virus in the trigeminal nerve, which may be precipitated by generalised illness/immunosuppression. Clinical features include as a classical tingling across the Vb distribution and severe pain in the eye. Treatment is with topical antivirals and dilating agents to prevent iris scarring. It is complicated by a high incidence of permanent visual loss.

- The table below provides a summary of eye infections:

Organisms	Examples	Presentation	Treatment
Bacteria	*Staphylococcus aureus*	Acute red eye. Honey-coloured discharge	Topical antibiotics
Other viruses	Adenovirus	Red watery eyes. May progress to keratitis	Topical aciclovir
Herpes	Herpes zoster, herpes simplex	Neuropathic pain in Va distribution. Visual loss	Antivirals. Dexamethasone (Maxidex, and Maxitrol)
CMV	Cytomegalovirus	Visual loss. 'Pizza pie' appearance	Specialist ophthalmological
Fungi	*Candida* spp.	Severe uveitis. Common in intravenous drug misusers	Specialist ophthalmological
Chlamydia	*Chlamydia*	Chronic unilateral conjunctivitis	Systemic tetracyclines

ORAL AND MAXILLOFACIAL SURGERY

136 THEME: CLASSIFICATION OF FACIAL FRACTURES

A   Dental fractures
B   Fractured mandible
C   Fractured zygomatic complex
D   LeFort I fracture
E   LeFort II fracture
F   LeFort III fracture
G   LeFort IV fracture
H   Nasal bone fracture
I   Panfacial fracture

From the list above, select the single most likely diagnosis for each of the following clinical scenarios. The items may be used once, more than once or not at all.

☐ 1   A 28-year-old woman is thrown from her horse, sustaining facial injuries. On arrival, her GCS score is 15/15. On examination, she has trismus, dental malocclusion and lower lip hypoaesthesia.

☐ 2   A 21-year-old man is an unrestrained passenger in a high-speed road traffic accident, sustaining severe head and facial injuries. On arrival at A&E his GCS score is 10/15. On examination, there is gross midfacial swelling and bilateral periorbital haematomata. Examination of the anterior nares reveals previous epistaxis and now evidence of clear fluid leakage. The maxillary segment is mobile on anterior traction.

☐ 3   A 36-year-old man is hit is the face with a baseball bat during an assault. On examination, his GCS score is 12/15. On examination, there is evidence of stridor. There is marked periorbital oedema bilaterally and evidence of infraorbital paraesthesia. There is an obvious nasal deformity with marked epistaxis and evidence of stepping of the infraorbital margin. In addition, there is dental malocclusion due to obvious dislocation at the temporomandibular joint.

136 CLASSIFICATION OF FACIAL FRACTURES

1** **B – Fractured mandible**
The three cardinal features of such fractures are described.

2** **F – LeFort III fracture**
This results in disjunction of the mid-facial skeleton from the cranial base.

3** **I – Panfacial fracture**
Features of nasal, zygomatic, maxillary and mandibular fractures are described.

• See ERN MRCS Book 1, Chapter 5, section 4.2 and ATLS student course manual.

• High-energy blunt force injury to the facial skeleton may result in fractures of the orbital walls, the nasoethmoidal and zygomatic complexes, the maxilla or the mandible.

• Maxillary fractures deserve special mention and are classified as follows:

   – LeFort I – fractures through horizontal buttress of maxilla.
   – LeFort II – fracture through horizontal buttress of **infra**orbital bones.
   – LeFort III – fracture through horizontal buttress of **supra**orbital ridge.

• The LeFort classification, which dates back to the early 1900s, is a simplification of the types of mid-face fractures seen in today's high-energy injuries where panfacial fractures are increasingly encountered.

137 THEME: MANAGEMENT OF FACIAL FRACTURES

A	Antibiotics and CT scan of the head
B	Closed reduction
C	Conservative management
D	Discharge
E	Internal suspension
F	Observation of neurological parameters
G	Open reduction and internal fixation
H	Rest, soft diet and analgesia

From the list above, select the single most appropriate next step in management in the following clinical scenarios. The items may be used once, more than once or not at all.

1 A 27-year-old man sustains a blow to the mandible during a fight. On examination, there is no mobility or malocclusion. 'Facial view' X-rays review a fracture of the angle of the mandible.

2 A 55-year-old homeless woman attends A&E with evidence of an injury to the face. The event was not witnessed and the patient is unable to provide any useful information due to alcohol intoxication. There is evidence of epistaxis. There is an obvious deformity of the nasal bone.

3 A 32-year-old man is involved in a collision playing rugby, sustaining facial injuries. On arrival his GCS score is 15/15. On examination, there is displacement of the midfacial segment and facial CT reveals a displaced LeFort I fracture of the right side of the maxilla.

137 MANAGEMENT OF FACIAL FRACTURES

1**   **H – Rest, soft diet and analgesia**

2   **B – Closed reduction**
Deformity can usually be treated with immediate closed reduction.
Otherwise, reduction/fixation can be undertaken under general
anaesthesia, usually 7–10 days later to allow reduction of soft-tissue
swelling.

3**   **G – Open reduction and internal fixation**

- See ERN MRCS Book 1, Chapter 5, section 4.2 and ATLS student course
  manual.

- It is important to remember that maxillofacial trauma can result in
  airway and circulatory compromise and injuries to the cervical spine and
  brain.

- Initial management, therefore, is in accordance with the principles of
  ATLS.

- CT scanning helps characterise the nature of the fracture.

- Rhinorrhoea may be due to cerebrospinal fluid (CSF) leak. This is usually
  managed conservatively but CT head is indicated. Antibiotics should be
  commenced as soon as breach of meninges is suspected.

- In general, undisplaced fractures without mobility or malocclusion are
  managed with rest, soft diet and analgesia. Otherwise open-reduction
  and internal fixation (ORIF) must be considered.

138 THEME: MANDIBULAR FRACTURES

A   Fracture of the angle of the mandible
B   Fracture of the body of the mandible
C   Fracture of the condyle of the mandible
D   Fracture of the ramus of the mandible
E   Panfacial fracture

From the list above, select the most appropriate answer for each of the following clinical scenarios. The items may be used once, more than once or not at all.

☐ 1   A young male patient presents with trismus after a blow to the side of the face. The jaw is not displaced but his face is grossly swollen. The radiologist reports the X-rays and informs you that the patient has sustained the most common type of mandibular fracture.

☐ 2   A 17-year-old patient attends A&E having sustained a direct blow to the jaw. On examination, there is no evidence of malocclusion but there is extreme pain on jaw opening. There is marked tenderness and swelling in preauricular region.

139 THEME: ORAL LESIONS

A   Aphthous ulceration
B   Dental abscess
C   Leucoplakia
D   Mucocoele
E   Pyogenic granuloma
F   Ranula
G   Squamous cell carcinoma
H   Sublingual dermoid
I   Thyroglossal cyst

From the list above, select the single most likely diagnosis for each of the following clinical scenarios described below. The items may be used once, more than once or not at all.

☐ 1   A 49-year-old woman is referred for assessment of a longstanding lump in her mouth. On examination, she has a 1-cm diameter blue–grey fluctuant domed-shaped swelling in the floor of her mouth.

☐ 2   A young man is found to have a midline swelling in the neck that has been present since birth. It moves on protrusion of the tongue.

☐ 3   A 27-year-old woman develops a swelling in the mouth. This is treated by surgical excision. The histological report is 'a mass of lymphocytes'.

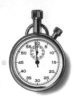

138 MANDIBULAR FRACTURES

1   **B – Fracture of the body of the mandible**

2**   **C – Fracture of the condyle of the mandible**

- See ERN MRCS Book 1, Chapter 5, section 4.2 and ATLS student course manual.

- Clinical findings of mandibular fractures include facial distortion, malocclusion of the teeth or abnormal mobility of portions of the mandible or teeth.

- Most fractures occur in the body, followed by the condyle and angle of the mandible.

- Fractures are usually adequately seen on plain X-ray.

- Traditionally, closed reduction and ORIF with wire osteosynthesis have required an average of 6 weeks of immobilization for satisfactory healing.

- ORIF has dramatically revolutionised the approach to mandibular fractures and avoids the problems encountered with intermaxillary fixation (airway problems, weight loss, poor hygiene, phonation difficulties, loss of range of jaw function).

139 ORAL LESIONS

1   **F – Ranula**

2**   **I – Thyroglossal cyst**

3   **E – Pyogenic granuloma**

- See ERN MRCS Book 2, Chapter 3, section 3.3.

- Examination of oral lesions is also commonly encountered in the clinical section (Part IV) of the Intercollegiate MRCS!

- Thyroglossal cysts occur in the midline and move with tongue excursion. They represent remnants of thyroglossal duct and can be treated by excision of the entire tract.

- Pyogenic granulomata are caused by an overproduction of granulation tissue in response to chronic infection or foreign bodies.

- A ranula is a mucus retention cyst, which occurs in the floor of the mouth. Excision is technically demanding as there is a risk of injury to the submandibular duct/lingual nerve and of recurrence if excision is incomplete.

140 THEME: HEAD AND NECK INFECTIONS

A	Candidiasis
B	Cavernous sinus thrombosis
C	Dental abscess
D	Glossitis
E	Ludwig's angina
F	Necrotising fasciitis
G	Parotitis
H	Tonsillar abscess

From the list above, select the single most likely diagnosis for each of the following clinical scenarios described below. The items may be used once, more than once or not at all.

1. A 27-year-old man attends A&E with a 6-day history of a swollen and red lesion in the infraorbital region. He now reports severe headache and fevers. On examination, he has a bulging left eye with evidence of diplopia.

2. A 26-year-old woman presents with difficulty in breathing and stridor. She has a history of impacted wisdom teeth. On examination, there is marked submandibular swelling and cervical lymphadenopathy.

141 THEME: MALIGNANT AND PREMALIGNANT LESIONS OF THE ORAL CAVITY

A	Basal cell carcinoma
B	Kaposi's sarcoma
C	Leiomyosarcoma
D	Leucoplakia
E	Melanoma
F	Rhabdomyosarcoma
G	Squamous cell carcinoma

From the list above, select the single most likely diagnosis for each of the following clinical scenarios described below. The items may be used once, more than once or not at all.

1. A 65-year-old man, who is a long-term smoker, is referred for assessment of a lesion on the inner aspect of the lower lip. On examination, there is a 3-cm diameter ulcerated lesion inside the lower lip. There is associated cervical lymphadenopathy.

2. You are asked to review a white lesion on the tongue of a 75-year-old man, who is admitted with acute lower abdominal pain 2 days ago. He tells you that it has been present for several months and that it was biopsied 2 months ago. A review of the histopathology result reveals moderate dysplasia.

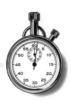

140 HEAD AND NECK INFECTIONS

1**   **B – Cavernous sinus thrombosis**

2   **E – Ludwig's angina**

- Infection of the oral cavity and face spreads via the bloodstream, lymphatics and, most importantly, along fascial planes.

- Spread of infection from the maxillary region via veins to the cavernous sinus may result in cavernous sinus thrombosis (ptosis, proptosis and ophthalmoplegia). Rarely, infection from the cavernous sinus may result in brain abscesses.

- Ludwig's angina results from bilateral infection of the submandibular, sublingual and submental spaces. Most arise from dental sepsis. The infection spreads rapidly along deep cervical and parapharyngeal fascial planes, potentially resulting in airways obstruction.

141 MALIGNANT AND PREMALIGNANT LESIONS OF THE ORAL CAVITY

1**   **G – Squamous cell carcinoma**

2   **D – Leucoplakia**

- See ERN MRCS Book 2, Chapter 3, section 3.3.

- Basal cell carcinoma is the commonest cancer of the head and neck. Treatment is with excision.

- Cancers of the mucosa of head and neck are generally squamous cell carcinomas.

- 85% of oral malignancies are squamous cell carcinomas. They tend to occur in the salivary gutters and risk factors include (the 's's): smoking, spirits (alcohol), sepsis, sharp tooth (recurrent trauma) and betel nut chewing.

- Tumours are staged using the TNM classification.

- Treatment involves surgery and/or radiotherapy to the primary lesion ± cervical lymph nodes.

- Leucoplakia is a premalignant lesion with stages of increasing dysplasia that can ultimately lead to squamous cell carcinoma.

PAEDIATRIC SURGERY

142 THEME: CONSENT IN CHILDREN

A   Adult sibling
B   Doctor
C   Foster carer
D   Grandparent without parental responsibility
E   Judge
F   Parent
G   Patient
H   Social services

From the list above select the person/people from whom consent should be sought in each of the scenarios described below. The items may be used once, more than once or not at all.

☐ 1   A newborn with necrotising enterocolitis is profoundly shocked. She needs an urgent laparotomy. The police have been unable to locate her parents and they are not answering their telephone.

☐ 2   You are working as an SHO in A&E when you see a 15-year-old girl who has had unprotected sexual intercourse. She is requesting a prescription for 'emergency contraception'.

☐ 3   A 4-year-old child is brought in by ambulance and is suspected of having appendicitis. She is in foster care while an investigation into suspected abuse of a sibling is being undertaken. Her parents retain parental responsibility.

142 CONSENT IN CHILDREN

1   B – Doctor

2   G – Patient

3**   F – Parent

- See ERN MRCS Book 1, Chapter 10, section 1.3.

- A person of 16 years or older can consent to treatment (although a person must be 18 years or over to decline treatment).

- A person under the age of 16 years **can** consent to intervention **if** they are judged to be competent (after the Gillick case).

- Below the age of 16 years, a person with parental responsibility may authorise investigation and/or treatment. This can be awarded to people other than the parents by the courts to social services, foster carers or adoptive parents.

- Refusal of intervention by those with parental responsibility may be challenged in the law courts.

- Doctors can make decisions to act in the best interests of the patient in life-threatening situations.

143 THEME: FLUID AND ELECTROLYTE BALANCE

A	10 ml/kg blood
B	20 ml/kg normal saline
C	40 ml/kg 4.5% human albumin
D	100 ml/kg/day 0.18% saline/4% dextrose
E	120 ml/kg/day 10% dextrose
F	200 ml/kg/day 0.18% saline/4% dextrose
G	Weight (kg) × 10 ml × percentage deficit
H	Weight (kg) × 100 ml × percentage deficit

From the list above select the most appropriate fluid regimen for each of the clinical scenarios described below. The items may be used once, more than once or not at all.

☐ 1 A 4-year-old child is brought in by ambulance following a road traffic accident with obvious lower limb fractures. On arrival, the child is tachycardic and hypotensive.

☐ 2 A 1-year-old infant, weighing 10 kg is admitted with tonsillitis. He is not taking any feed by mouth. The nursing staff ask you to prescribe maintenance fluids.

☐ 3 You admit a 4-year-old boy with lower abdominal pain. As a consequence of his associated diarrhoea and vomiting he is severely dehydrated. You are asked to prescribe appropriate fluids.

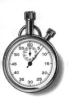

143 FLUID AND ELECTROLYTE BALANCE

1   B – 20 ml/kg normal saline

2   D – 100 ml/kg/day 0.18 saline/4% dextrose

3   G – Weight (kg) × 10 ml × percentage deficit

- See ERN MRCS Book 1, Chapter 10, section 1.3, ATLS student course manual and *BNF for Children*.

- ATLS guidelines for resuscitation of children:
  - – initially: 20 ml/kg normal saline
  - – then: 20 ml/kg normal saline
  - – then: 10 ml/kg blood.

- Maintenance fluids:
  - – First 10 kg bodyweight: 100ml/kg/day.
  - – For next 10 kg up to 20 kg bodyweight add 50 ml/kg/day.
  - – For each kilogram over 20 kg add 20 ml/kg/day.
  - – Usually 0.18% saline/4% dextrose or 0.45% saline/5% dextrose is employed (depending on electrolyte measurement). 10% dextrose used in newborn who have higher glucose requirements and low glucose stores.

- Deficit replacement over 24 hours in addition to maintenance fluid:
  - – Amount of fluid (ml) = weight (kg) × 10 × percentage deficit.
  - – Percentage deficit is calculated from weight change or estimated based on clinical signs.

144 THEME: VASCULAR ACCESS IN CHILDREN

A   Hickman's line
B   Intraosseous needle
C   Peripheral inserted central catheter (PICC line)
D   Peripheral venous catheter
E   Fogarty's catheter
F   Umbilical artery catheter
G   Umbilical venous catheter

From the list above, select the single most appropriate means of vascular access for each of the clinical scenarios described below. The items may be used once, more than once or not at all.

1   A 3-year-old girl is in resuscitation in A&E following a road traffic accident. She is severely shocked with 'peripheral shutdown'. Cannulation has failed on three attempts.

2   A 5-year-old girl is being treated with chemotherapy for nephroblastoma. Long-term venous sampling and iv drug administration are required. Her mother has requested that the child be allowed to bathe normally.

3   A newborn has had large segments of bowel resected for necrotising enterocolitis. She requires repeated iv administration of medications and fluids, including total parenteral nutrition.

145 THEME: CONGENITAL ABNORMALITIES OF THE GASTROINTESTINAL TRACT

A   Duodenal atresia
B   Hirschsprung's disease
C   Imperforate anus
D   Malrotation
E   Meckel's diverticulum
F   Diverticular disease
G   Pharyngeal pouch
H   Tracheo-oesophageal fistula (H-type)

From the list above, select the single most likely diagnosis in each of the following clinical scenarios. The items may be used once, more than once or not at all.

1   A 4-day-old baby boy is noted to have increasing abdominal distension. On questioning his mother, it transpires that there has been no meconium/stool passed per anum since birth. On examination, there is gross abdominal distension and increased bowel sounds.

2   A 1-week-old baby with antenatal diagnosis of Down's syndrome presents with bilious vomiting without abdominal distension.

144 VASCULAR ACCESS IN CHILDREN

1   B – Intraosseous needle

2   A – Hickman's line

3**   G – Umbilical venous catheter

- See ERN MRCS Book 1, Chapter 10, section 1.3 and the ATLS student course manual.

- Intraosseous needles can be used in children < 6 years. Care must be taken not to injure the growth plate on insertion. Any medication or fluid can be administered except bretylium.

- Hickman's lines are a means of central venous access that are tunnelled underneath the skin into the large veins of the neck.

- Umbilical venous and artery catheters can only be used in newborns while umbilical vessels are patent. Umbilical venous catheter is for fluids and medication administration. Umbilical artery catheter is used for invasive BP and arterial blood gases monitoring (cf arterial lines).

145 CONGENITAL ABNORMALITIES OF THE GASTROINTESTINAL TRACT

1**   B – Hirschsprung's disease

2   A – Duodenal atresia

- See ERN MRCS Book 1, Chapter 10, section 2.1.

- Hirschsprung's disease results from a hypoganglionic/aganglionic segment of distal anorectum. As a consequence of failure of relaxation, a functional obstruction occurs leading to constipation, abdominal distension and vomiting. Diagnosis is confirmed on histological analysis of full-thickness anorectal biopsy. Treatment is by laparotomy and pull through (Duhamel's procedure).

- 30% of patients with duodenal atresia have Down's syndrome. Presentation is with high obstruction. The second part of the duodenum is the commonest site of atresia.

146 THEME: CONGENITAL ABNORMALITIES

A   Appendix of Morgagni
B   Bladder exstrophy
C   Diaphragmatic hernia – Bochdalek's type
D   Diaphragmatic hernia – Morgagni's type
E   Exomphalos
F   Gastroschisis
G   Indirect inguinal hernia
H   Meconium aspiration
I   Thyroglossal cyst

From the list above, select the single most likely diagnosis in each of the clinical scenarios described below. The items may be used once, more than once or not at all.

☐ 1   A newborn develops respiratory distress immediately after birth and requires ventilation. Chest X-ray reveals a large opacity affecting the inferior aspect of the right hemi-thorax.

☐ 2   A newborn is delivered by elective Caesarean section with its abdominal contents herniating through a defect in the abdominal wall. The umbilicus appears normal.

☐ 3   A baby is born with its abdominal viscera protruding through the base of the umbilicus, covered with amniotic sac.

146 CONGENITAL ABNORMALITIES

1   **C – Diaphragmatic hernia – Bochdalek's type**

2**   **F – Gastroschisis**

3**   **E – Exomphalos**

- See ERN MRCS Book 1, Chapter 10, sections 2 and 3.

- Diaphragmatic herniae allow abdominal contents to enter the thorax. This may compromise the development of the lungs, resulting in pulmonary hypoplasia. There are two types:

  - posterolateral (Bochdalek) large defect
  - anterior (Morgagni) often asymptomatic.

- Exomphalos describes herniation of abdominal contents into the base of the umbilical cord. The abdominal viscera are thus covered by a (amniotic) sac. It is associated with increased risk of renal and cardiac abnormalities.

- Gastroschisis describes herniation of abdominal contents through defect in abdominal wall but lateral to the umbilicus. As there is no covering, immediate protection with cling film is required. There is an increased risk of bowel atresia.

147 THEME: GASTROINTESTINAL BLEEDING IN CHILDREN

A	Haemorrhagic disease of the newborn
B	Henoch–Schönlein's purpura
C	Intussusception
D	Meckel's diverticulum
E	Necrotising enterocolitis (NEC)
F	Pyloric stenosis
G	von Willenbrand's disease

From the list above, select the single most likely diagnosis for each of the clinical scenarios described below. The items may be used once, more than once or not at all.

1 A 6-month-old child is brought to A&E with acute colicky abdominal pain and vomiting. In the department the child passes a red stool. On examination, the abdomen is distended but generally soft.

2 A 12-day-old child born at 28 weeks' gestation develops a distended abdomen. The child is septic and peripherally shut down. There are features of peritonitis present on palpation of the abdomen.

3 A 12-week-old baby develops profuse non-bilious vomiting. His mother is alarmed to see the presence of fresh blood in the vomitus.

147 GASTROINTESTINAL BLEEDING IN CHILDREN

1   C – Intussusception

2   E – NEC

3**   F – Pyloric stenosis

- See ERN MRCS Book 1, Chapter 10, sections 2.1, 5.1 and 5.5.

- Intussusception – 90% idiopathic, 10% have an abnormality (eg Meckel's etc) lesion at the leading edge. Infants present age 7–12 months with colicky abdominal pain (typical knees drawn to chest position) and vomiting. Up to 50% pass redcurrant jelly stools.

- NEC is an acute inflammatory condition of the neonatal bowel that may be associated with bowel necrosis and systemic inflammatory response syndrome. It is more common in premature babies. Necrosis of bowel results in an acute abdomen with signs of peritonitis. Plain abdominal X-ray shows air in bowel wall ± perforation. Treatment is with nasogastric tube and iv fluids, ventilatory support and correction of acidosis, with resection of necrotic bowel.

- Pyloric stenosis occurs secondary to hypertrophy and hyperplasia of the muscular layers of the pylorus, causing a functional gastric outlet obstruction. Classically, the infant will have non-bilious vomiting, which may become projectile. The vomitus may contain fresh red blood or become brown or coffee grounds due to the development of blood secondary to a Mallory–Weiss tear or gastritis, respectively.

- Meckel's diverticulum – ectopic gastric mucosa, usually asymptomatic. Can ulcerate and perforate. Usually presents with pain in the right iliac fossa, anaemia or the passage of brick red stools. Rarely, presentation is with massive lower gastrointestinal haemorrhage.

PLASTIC AND RECONSTRUCTIVE SURGERY

148 THEME: ASSESSMENT OF BURNS

A	4.5% deep dermal
B	4.5% full thickness
C	4.5% superficial
D	9% deep dermal
E	9% full thickness
F	9% superficial
G	10% deep dermal
H	10% full thickness
I	10% superficial
J	18% deep dermal
K	18% full thickness
L	18% superficial

From the list above select the single most appropriate option for the most accurate assessment of the burn described in each of the following clinical scenarios. The items may be used once, more than once or not at all.

1 A gas engineer presents to the burns unit following a blast injury. He has painful sensate burns with blistering covering the whole of the anterior and posterior aspect of his right arm and hand.

2 An elderly woman is caught in a house fire and receives burns to both lower legs to the knee. She is surprisingly comfortable and requires minimal analgesia.

3 A 7-year-old boy presents to casualty after he pulled a recently boiled kettle from a work top on to himself. Approximately half of his anterior torso is erythematous and acutely painful.

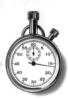

1**   **G – 10% deep dermal**
       (ie partial thickness burns)

2   **K – 18% full thickness**

3   **F – 9% superficial**

- See ERN MRCS Book 1, Chapter 5, section 2.1.

- Wallace's rule of '9's allows estimation of the area of the burn – head: 9%; arms: 9% each; palms: 1% each; thorax and abdomen front: 18%; thorax and abdomen back: 18%; lower limb: 18% each (9% anterior, 9% posterior surface); perineum: 1%.

- 15% and 10% area constitutes major burns in adults and children, respectively.

- Immediate consequences include: hypovolaemia, increased haematocrit, metabolism and cortisol levels.

- The table shows some features of burns of different depths:

Cause	Degree/depth	Appearance	Pain
Hot liquids/steam	Superficial	Erythema	Painful
Flames/hot liquids	Partial thickness	Red/blistered	Painful
Chemicals/electricity oil/flames	Full thickness	Dry/waxy White/red mottled	Insensate

149 THEME: COMPLICATIONS OF BURNS

A	Compartment syndrome
B	Curling's ulcer
C	Eschar formation
D	Hypovolaemia and shock
E	Infection
F	Joint contractures
G	Rhabdomyolysis and renal failure
H	Smoke inhalation and airway oedema

From the list above select the single most likely diagnosis for each of the following clinical scenarios. The items may be used once, more than once or not at all.

1 A 38-year-old woman wakes in the night to a smoke-filled bedroom. She is trapped for 20 minutes before emergency services can rescue her. She suffers full thickness burns to the soles of her feet and is seen to have singed eyebrows and soot around the nostrils.

2 A 78-year-old woman, who weighs 75 kg, falls to the floor pulling a pan full of boiling chip fat over herself. She sustains 16% mixed deep dermal and full thickness burns. She is unable to call for help and is on the floor for 6 hours before being found by her neighbour. She receives 4800 ml of fluid in the first 24 hours following admission.

3 A 23-year-old electrician sustains an electrical burn at work while standing on a wet floor. He has entry and exit wound on the left foot and buttock, respectively. Despite sustaining less than 9% total burns, he is complaining of disproportionate pain throughout his left leg.

4 A 100 kg man presents to casualty with 15% partial thickness burns to his torso and shoulder. None of which are circumferential. He has his burns dressed with a sterile dressing and is given 5000 ml fluid in the first 24 hours following admission.

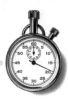

149 COMPLICATIONS OF BURNS

1   H – Smoke inhalation and airway oedema

2   G – Rhabdomyolysis and renal failure

3   A – Compartment syndrome

4**   D – Hypovolaemia and shock
Inadequate fluid replacement – closer to 6 litres is required.

- See ERN MRCS Book 1, Chapter 5, section 2.1.

- Remember smoke inhalation is diagnosed through history, singed facial hair, carbonaceous sputum, shortness of breath and soot surrounding the nose and mouth. The airway is at significant risk in such patients.

- Having secured the airway and breathing, the priority of management is to prevent hypovolaemia and its potential consequences. Many formulae are available to calculate fluid requirements (eg Mount Vernon/Brooke Army Hospital).

- Rhabdomyolysis is an important cause of morbidity and mortality in burns victims, as well as following long periods of lying immobilised.

- Compartment syndrome may occur secondary to any burn to the limbs but is highly likely following an electrical burn, as the current passes preferentially through the vessels causing major injury and rapid limb oedema.

- Eschar formation may result in loss of a limb, joint contraction and even respiratory failure. Urgent escharotomy must be performed.

150 THEME: DISORDERS OF THE HAND AND WRIST

A   Carpal tunnel syndrome
B   Compartment syndrome
C   De Quervain's syndrome
D   Dupuytren's disease
E   Extensor tendon rupture
F   Kienböck's disease
G   Reflex sympathetic dystrophy
H   Tenovaginitis stenosans (trigger finger)

From the list above, select the single most likely diagnosis for each of the following clinical scenarios. The items may be used once, more than once or not at all.

☐ 1 A 78-year-old woman presents to the outpatient clinic holding her hand in an unusual manner. She gives no recent history of trauma, and does not apparently have any new acute problems. She reports a fall 6 months ago, following which she did not seek medical attention. On examination, she is unable to extend the thumb.

☐ 2 A 39-year-old pregnant woman presents with a sudden onset of shooting pains in the hand. They keep her up at night and appear to be localised to the radial two fingers and the thumb. She has also recently noticed difficulty with precision grip.

☐ 3 A young man presents to fracture clinic with sudden onset of pain in the dorsum of the wrist. He gives no history of trauma. Examination of the wrist reveals only mild tenderness over the dorsum. X-ray of the wrist shows a hyperlucency at the base of the lunate bone.

150 DISORDERS OF THE HAND AND WRIST

1   E – Extensor tendon rupture

2   A – Carpal tunnel syndrome

3**   F – Kienböck's disease
        Typical presentation described.

•   See ERN MRCS Book 2, Chapter 2, sections 3.14–3.16.

•   Examination of disorders of the hand and wrist is commonly
        encountered in the clinical section (Part IV) of the Intercollegiate MRCS!

•   Extensor pollicis longus rupture is common 3–6 months following an
        undisplaced distal radius fracture.

•   Carpal tunnel syndrome is the most common compressive neuropathy.
        Features include shooting pains down the medial two and half fingers,
        exacerbation of symptoms at night. Thenar wasting and median nerve
        dysfunction may be evident on examination. Other compressive
        neuropathies such as tarsal tunnel syndrome and cubital tunnel
        syndrome are also well described.

•   Keinböck's disease is avascular necrosis of the lunate, a relatively
        uncommon condition that invariably demands surgical intervention.

151 THEME: PRINCIPLES OF SKIN COVER

A	Deep tension sutures
B	Free flap
C	Full thickness skin graft
D	Pedicled flap
E	Rotational flap
F	Split skin graft
G	Undermine margins
H	V–Y plasty
I	Z plasty

From the list above, select the single most appropriate method of skin cover for each of the following clinical scenarios. The items may be used once, more than once or not at all.

1 A 60-year-old male undergoes dermofasciectomy for Dupuytren's disease, leaving a large deficit on the volar aspect of the hand and index/middle fingers.

2 A 17-year-old woman amputates the distal pulp of her finger with a cooking knife. There is no bony injury, but the soft tissues cannot be opposed.

3 After removing a skin lump under local anaesthetic from the back of a patient the skin is under tension when closure is attempted.

151 PRINCIPLES OF SKIN COVER

1   **F – Split skin graft**

2**   **H – V–Y plasty**

3   **G – Undermine margins**

- See ERN MRCS Book 1, Chapter 1, section 3.3.

- **Wound closure** is done in stages when difficult:

  1   Carefully place incision to ensure soft tissue coverage.

  2   Undermine edges.

  3   Deep tension or tension sutures.

- **Plasty** such as V–Y (advancement) or Z (sacrificing length for breadth) can cover a deficit by sacrificing length for width.

  Flaps and skin grafts
- **Flaps** are used to cover large deficits with skin and soft tissue. Examples include latissimus dorsi flap (pedicled) and TRAM (trans-rectus abdominis muscle; free). They consist not only of skin but also of connective tissue and sometimes muscle and have their **own blood supply**.

- **Grafts** contain only skin and are used to cover large deficits or to transpose disease free skin (such as in Dupuytren's disease). They are either split skin (partial thickness) or full thickness.

152 THEME: BENIGN SKIN CONDITIONS

A	Bowen's disease
B	Dermoid cyst
C	Ganglion
D	Keratoacanthoma
E	Lipoma
F	Pyogenic granuloma
G	Sebaceous cyst
H	Seborrhoeic warts

From the list above select the single most likely diagnosis for each of the following clinical scenarios. The items may be used once, more than once or not at all.

☐ 1 A 53-year-old gardener presents to the outpatient clinic with a small palpable lesion in the pulp of the right index finger. On examination, there is a 4-mm firm lesion in the pulp of the finger. Careful questioning reveals a history of trauma from a rose thorn 6 months previously.

☐ 2 A 76-year-old man is brought to clinic by his daughter who is concerned by a large number of heavily pigmented fleshy lesions that have appeared on her father's back. Although highly pigmented and spreading, there is no history of bleeding or change in pigmentation. On examination, the fleshy lesions are easily peeled off.

☐ 3 A 27-year-old man is referred by his GP with a large inflamed lesion on his shoulder. Between the initial referral and appointment, this has ruptured and left a small scar. There is a small palpable lesion underlying a scar, which has a central punctum and is within the skin.

152 BENIGN SKIN CONDITIONS

1**   B – Dermoid cyst

2   H – Seborrhoeic warts

3   G – Sebaceous cyst

- See ERN MRCS Book 1, Chapter 1, section 4.1.

- Another firm favourite of examiners of the clinical section (Part IV) of the Intercollegiate MRCS!

- Dermoid cysts may be congenital (commonly in the lines of embryonic fusion) or acquired (implantation). An implantation dermoid occurs following injury when a remnant of dermis is driven into the subdermal layer.

- Seborrhoeic warts represent a benign overgrowth of the basal layer of the epidermis. Their classic features are described.

- Sebaceous cysts are found *within* the skin (which thus cannot be drawn across them) and contain a central punctum. They may become inflamed and infected. In contrast, lipomas are under the skin (which can thus be drawn across them), are usually soft and may be attached to underlying structures (eg muscle). Clearly, they do not have a punctum.

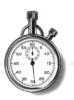

153 THEME: STAGING OF CUTANEOUS MALIGNANCY

A	Clark level I
B	Clark level II
C	Clark level III
D	Clark level IV
E	Clark level V
F	$T_1 N_1 M_0$
G	$T_2 N_1 M_0$
H	$T_3 N_1 M_0$
I	$T_4 N_1 M_0$
J	$T_1 N_2 M_0$
K	$T_3 N_2 M_1$

From the list above, select the single most appropriate description of the lesions in each of the following scenarios. The items may be used once, more than once or not at all.

1 A large nodular malignant melanoma is excised together with its draining lymph nodes. The lesion is found to be 5 mm in depth, and a single local lymph node is involved.

2 A young man presents to the outpatient clinic with a single superficial spreading malignant melanoma. Examination reveals a satellite lesion.

3 A single acral malignant melanoma is completely excised and found to extend throughout the papillary dermis.

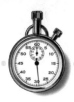

153 STAGING OF CUTANEOUS MALIGNANCY

1   I – $T_4 N_1 M_0$

2**   K – $T_3 N_2 M_1$
      The tumour has metastasised.

3   **C – Clark level III**

•   See ERN MRCS Book 1, Chapter 1, section 4.7.

•   Breslow's thickness measures the depth of the lesion (ie from the top of the tumour to the deepest area of spread). It correlates to prognosis (5-year survival: < 0.75 mm = 97%; 0.75–1.5 mm = 93%; 1.5–3.49 mm = 67%; > 3.5 mm = 37%).

•   Breslow's thickness also forms the basis of the TNM classification for malignant melanoma:

     T_1 < 1 mm (comparable to Clark level II)
     T_2 1–2 mm (comparable to Clark level III)
     T_3 2–4 mm (comparable to Clark level IV)
     T_4 > 4 mm (comparable to Clark level V)

•   Clark levels:

     I – Confined to epidermis
     II – Invasion into upper papillary dermis
     III – Invasion into papillary dermis
     IV – Invasion into reticular dermis
     V – Invasion into subcutaneous fat

154 THEME: TREATMENT FOR CUTANEOUS MALIGNANCY

A	En-bloc dissection of regional lymph nodes
B	Local excision
C	Local excision + chemotherapy
D	Local excision + radiotherapy
E	Local excision + sentinel node biopsy
F	Localised radiotherapy
G	Systemic chemotherapy only

From the list above, select the single most appropriate treatment option for the following clinical scenarios. The items may be used once, more than once or not at all.

1 A 78-year-old man presents with an advanced squamous cell carcinoma involving the ear and cheek, which appears to be 'full thickness'.

2 A 37-year-old man presents with a small malignant melanoma of the ciliary body.

3 A 78-year-old man presents with a rodent ulcer involving 30% of the anterior surface of the nose.

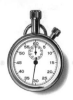

154 TREATMENT FOR CUTANEOUS MALIGNANCY

1   **F – Localised radiotherapy**

2** **F – Localised radiotherapy**

3   **B – Local excision**

- See ERN MRCS Book 1, Chapter 1, section 4.7.

- Squamous cell carcinomas respond well to external beam radiotherapy. In advanced cases or irresectable cases the tumour may shrink to a size manageable surgically, or even provide definitive treatment.

- Although normally radio-resistant, melanoma of the ciliary body and iris may be effectively treated with localised radiotherapy.

- Local excision forms the mainstay of treatment for basal cell carcinomas, as, although locally invasive and destructive, metastatic disease is extremely rare.

- Management of malignant melanoma comprises treatment of the primary tumour (surgical excision with 5–30 mm margin depending on T stage) and treatment of regional lymph nodes (en-bloc dissection is indicated following FNAC confirmation of involvement). Currently, sentinel lymph node biopsy remains controversial and is not yet an accepted technique for any grade or stage of melanoma. The evidence from the literature suggests that in the future it is likely to become accepted in melanomas of > 1 mm or in recurrent tumours.

155 THEME: WOUND HEALING

A	Delayed primary intention (tertiary intent)
B	Epithelialisation
C	Hypertrophic scar formation
D	Keloid scar formation
E	Primary intention
F	Secondary intention

From the list above, select the single most appropriate type of healing described in each of the following clinical scenarios. The items may be used once, more than once or not at all.

1   A 47-year-old man undergoes a split skin graft procedure following excision of a large lesion on his finger. The donor site is left to heal.

2   A 17-year-old girl falls from her horse and sustains a compound tibia and fibula fracture. She undergoes surgical debridement. Initially, and the wound is left open prior to planned definitive closure.

3   A 76-year-old undergoes a laparotomy and Hartmann's procedure for an obstructing carcinoma in the sigmoid. Several days later, the patient develops a superficial wound dehiscence.

155 WOUND HEALING

1**   **B – Epithelialisation**

2   **A – Delayed primary intention (tertiary intent)**

3   **F – Secondary intention**

- See ERN MRCS Book 1, Chapter 1, section 1.3.

- The traditional types of healing are:

    - **Primary**: when a wound heals edge to edge.
    - **Secondary**: when a wound granulates from the base.
    - **Tertiary** (or delayed primary): when an infected wound is left open prior to definitive closure, eg infected wounds.

- Epithelialisation (strictly a subtype of secondary intent) occurs from the dermis when partial thickness deficits are present, eg following split skin grafting.

- Common forms of incomplete resolution include:

    - **Keloid** scarring – extends beyond the limits of the wound.
    - **Hypertrophic** scarring – does **not** extend beyond the original wound edges.

NEUROSURGERY

156 THEME: HEAD INJURY MANAGEMENT

A	Admit for neurological observation
B	Cervical spine X-ray
C	CT scan of head
D	CT scan of head and cervical spine X-ray
E	Discharge with head injury advice sheet
F	Emergency burr hole
G	Endotracheal intubation
H	Immediate laparotomy
I	Intracranial pressuremonitoring
J	iv mannitol
K	iv steroids
L	MRI of the brain
M	MRI of the spine
N	Skull X-ray

From the list above select the single most appropriate next step in management for each of the following clinical scenarios. The items may be used once, more than once or not at all.

1 A 64-year-old woman, who is living alone, is brought to A&E after falling down the stairs at her home. There appears to have been a brief loss of consciousness following the fall. She has a history of recurrent pulmonary embolism for which she is on warfarin. On examination, her GCS score is 15/15. There is no cervical spine tenderness and there is full range of movements. There are no injuries apart from a 1-cm superficial laceration on the forehead.

2 An 18-year-old motorcyclist is brought to A&E after being hit from behind by a lorry at high speed on the motorway. His GCS score on the scene when the paramedics arrived was 13/15. A trauma call was sent out due to the high velocity of the collision. On arrival, his GCS score drops to 7/15 and his right pupil is fixed and dilated.

3 An 8-year-old boy is brought to A&E by his mother after falling from his bike and sustaining a head injury. There was no loss of consciousness. He vomited once immediately after the fall. On examination his GCS score is 15/15. A small scalp laceration that was present was glued. There are no other injuries.

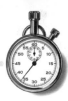

156 HEAD INJURY MANAGEMENT

1** **C – CT scan of the head**

2 **G – Endotracheal intubation**

3 **E – Discharge with head injury advice sheet**

- See ERN MRCS Book 1, Chapter 5, section 4.2, ATLS student course manual and NICE, *Head injury: triage, assessment, investigation and early management of head injury in infants, children and adults*, London: NICE, 2003 (www.nice.org.uk/page.aspx?o=CG004).

- Essentially, NICE and the Canadian Head CT guidelines recommend an urgent CT (< 1 hour) when: (i) GCS score < 13 at any point since injury; (ii) GCS score 13 or 14 with failure to regain GCS score 15 within 2 hours; (iii) suspected open or depressed skull fracture; (iv) any sign of basal skull fracture (Battle's sign, haemotympanum etc); (v) > 1 episode of vomiting; (vi) retrograde amnesia of > 30 minutes; (vii) post-traumatic seizure; or (viii) focal neurological deficit.

- In addition, the following require CT if accompanied with loss of consciousness or amnesia: (i) age > 64 years; (ii) coagulopathy (including anticoagulant therapy); or (iii) dangerous mechanism of injury (pedestrian hit by vehicle, fall from a height etc).

- GCS score < 8 intubate immediately.

157 THEME: BRAIN STEM DEATH

A   Confirmation of brain stem death
B   Exclusion of brain stem death
C   Need confirmatory tests of brain stem death
D   Repeat testing to confirm brain stem death

From the list above select the single most appropriate conclusion for each of the following clinical scenarios. The items may be used once, more than once or not at all.

1   The ICU consultant conducts tests for brainstem death on a 24-year-old woman who was admitted with multiple injuries 3 weeks ago. Her temperature is 37 °C. Her electrolytes and arterial blood gases are within normal limits. On examination, there is no motor response to painful stimulus and all brainstem reflexes are absent. There is absence of spontaneous respiration at a $p_a(CO_2)$ of 38 mmHg.

2   The neurosurgical team decides to conduct testing for brain stem death on a 38-year-old man admitted to ICU 4 weeks ago with diffuse axonal injury. There are no electrolyte imbalances or acid base disorders. The body temperature is 30.6 °C. On examination, there is absent motor response to painful stimulus and all brainstem reflexes are absent. After disconnecting from the ventilator there is absence of spontaneous breathing effort at a $p_a(CO_2)$ of 60 mm Hg.

3   The neurology consultant is called to test for brainstem death on a 45-year-old man admitted to ICU for the past 2 weeks after a massive subarachnoid haemorrhage. There are no concurrent medical abnormalities. Arterial blood gases and electrolytes are normal. On examination, there is absent motor response to painful stimulus and all brainstem reflexes are absent. After disconnecting from the ventilator there is absence of spontaneous breathing effort at a $p_a(CO_2)$ of 60 mmHg.

157 BRAIN STEM DEATH

1   **D – Repeat testing to confirm brain stem death**

2**   **D – Repeat testing to confirm brain stem death**

3   **A – Confirmation of brain stem death**

- Apnoea should be tested at $p_a(CO_2) > 60$ mmHg to confirm brain death.

- Brainstem tests should not be interpreted in the presence of hypothermia (core temperature <32 °C), abnormal electrolytes and blood gases.

- Additional, confirmatory tests are optional in adults but **not** in children.

158 THEME: INTRACRANIAL HAEMORRHAGE

A	Acute subdural haematoma
B	Chronic subdural haematoma
C	Extradural haematoma
D	Intracerebral haematoma
E	Intraventricular haemorrhage
F	Subarachnoid haemorrhage

From the list above select the single most appropriate diagnosis for the following clinical scenarios. The items may be used once, more than once or not at all.

1   An 80-year-old nursing home resident is brought to A&E with a 2-day history of headache, drowsiness and gradually worsening right-sided weakness. Her carer says that she had a fall 2 weeks ago. There was no loss of consciousness at the time of the fall.

2   A 35-year-old man is brought to A&E having collapsed at home after a sudden episode of severe headache. He has a history of polycystic kidney disease. His blood pressure is 160/100 mmHg, heart rate is 50 bpm and his GCS score is 9/15.

3   A 40-year-old motorist is brought to A&E having been involved in a road traffic accident. On arrival, his GCS score is 8/15 and the left pupil is fixed and dilated. The paramedic crew who brought him to casualty say that he was fully conscious on scene but had a period of unconsciousness from which he recovered during transfer.

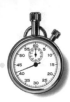

158 INTRACRANIAL HAEMORRHAGE

1   B – Chronic subdural haematoma

2**   F – Subarachnoid haemorrhage

3   C – Extradural haematoma

- See ERN MRCS Book 2, Chapter 6, section 1.3.

- Chronic subdural haematomata usually present a couple of weeks following trauma and are especially seen in elderly people.

- Acute onset, severe headache with loss of consciousness should raise the suspicion of subarachnoid haemorrhage. Hypertension, smoking, polycystic kidney disease are associated with rupture.

- The presence of a lucid interval and signs of raised intracranial pressure are characteristic of extradural haematomas.

159 THEME: SPINAL CORD INJURY

A	Anterior cord syndrome
B	Brown–Sequard syndrome
C	Central cord syndrome
D	Complete spinal cord injury
E	Incomplete spinal cord injury
F	Neurogenic shock
G	Spinal shock

From the list above select the single most appropriate diagnosis for the following clinical scenarios. The items may be used once, more than once or not at all.

1 A 64-year-old woman with a known history of cervical spondylosis is brought to A&E following a road traffic accident where she sustained a hyper-extension injury to her neck. Neurological examination reveals severe bilateral weakness in the upper limb, especially affecting the muscles of the hand. There is also mild weakness in both lower limbs. There is some loss of sensation in the cervical dermatomes although sacral sensation is intact.

2 A 28-year-old man is brought to A&E after falling from a height of 12 metres (40 feet). On arrival, he is breathing spontaneously and air entry is equal on both sides of the chest. His heart rate is 48 beats/min and blood pressure is 90/50 mmHg. He complains of pain between his shoulder blades.

3 A 28-year-old woman is brought to A&E following a bad landing during a parachute jump. On examination, her vital signs are stable. Neurological examination reveals a complete absence of sensory and motor function below bone T10. Rectal examination reveals normal voluntary contraction of the external sphincter.

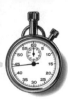

159 SPINAL CORD INJURY

1** C – Central cord syndrome

2 F – Neurogenic shock

3 E – Incomplete spinal cord injury

- See ERN MRCS Book 1, Chapter 5, section 4.6.

- In central cord syndrome, impairment of the upper extremity is usually greater than the lower. Sacral sensation is usually intact.

- Neurogenic shock usually occurs following cervical or high thoracic injuries. It is characterised by hypotension and bradycardia secondary to disruption of sympathetic pathways and unopposed vagal action.

- Rectal examination is essential as normal sphincter contraction and sensation may be the only preserved sacral cord functions. It helps to classify injuries into complete and incomplete.

160 THEME: INTRACRANIAL TUMOURS

A   Astrocytoma
B   Craniopharyngioma
C   Ependymoma
D   Glioblastoma multiforme
E   Medulloblastoma
F   Meningioma
G   Oligodendroglioma
H   Primary central nervous system lymphoma
I   Prolactinoma
J   Schwannoma
K   Secondary tumour

From the list above select the single most appropriate diagnosis for the following clinical scenarios. The items may be used once, more than once or not at all.

1   A 55-year-old man presents to A&E with a 3-week history of seizures and headache. He is due to see the respiratory physician for haemoptysis and weight loss.

2   A 70-year-old demented man had a fall and was brought A&E as he had a brief episode of loss of consciousness. A CT scan of his head reveals an enhancing extra-axial mass arising from the falx cerebri. There are no signs of intracranial haemorrhage.

3   A 68-year-old man presents to the ENT clinic with a 4-month history of right-sided, unilateral, progressive hearing loss. He has no other symptoms. On examination, he has weakness in the lower half of the right face.

4   A 45-year-old woman, who is HIV positive, complains of recurrent headaches. Neurological examination was unremarkable. A CT scan shows multiple ring-enhancing lesions.

160 INTRACRANIAL TUMOURS

1   **K – Secondary tumour**

2   **F – Meningioma**

3   **J – Schwannoma**

4**   **H – Primary CNS lymphoma**

- See ERN MRCS Book 2, Chapter 6, section 1.4.

- Secondaries are the commonest brain tumours.

- Meningiomas can be asymptomatic and can be may be visualised as an incidental finding.

- An acoustic neuroma is a type of schwannoma.

- Primary lymphoma of the central nervous system is common in immunocompromised patients.

161 THEME: INFECTIONS OF THE BRAIN AND SKULL

A   Brain abscess
B   Encephalitis
C   Epidural abscess
D   Meningitis
E   Osteomyelitis of skull
F   Septic cavernous sinus thrombosis
G   Subdural empyema

From the list above pick the single most appropriate diagnosis for the following clinical scenarios. The items may be used once, more than once or not at all.

1   A 28-year-old man with a history of recurrent middle ear infection and mastoiditis presents to A&E with severe headache and seizures. On examination, there is upper quadrant hemianopia. The diagnosis is confirmed on CT scan.

2   A 24-year-old man is brought to A&E with an altered level of consciousness, fever and right-sided weakness. He has a history of recurrent frontal sinusitis and has been complaining of a severe headache for the past 3 days.

3   A 30-year-old woman is brought to A&E with a 2-day history of headache, retro-orbital pain and diplopia. She is known to have recurrent attacks of pansinusitis. On examination, there is proptosis, ptosis and extraocular dysmotility. Examination of the fundus reveals dilated, tortuous retinal veins and papilloedema.

161 INFECTIONS OF THE BRAIN AND SKULL

1   A – Brain abscess

2**   G – Subdural empyema

3**   F – Septic cavernous sinus thrombosis

- See ERN MRCS Book 2, Chapter 6, section 1.7.

- Headache and seizures in the presence of mastoiditis should raise the suspicion of a temporal abscess. Upper quadrant hemianopia is a (true) localising sign.

- Hemiparesis is secondary to 'mass effect' and cortical venous thrombosis in subdural empyema

- Cavernous sinus thrombosis is a dangerous complication of facial sepsis. The presence of III, IV and VI cranial nerve palsies together with headache and proptosis is diagnostic.

TRAUMA AND ORTHOPAEDIC SURGERY

162 THEME: CLASSIFICATION OF FRACTURES

A	Avulsion
B	Comminuted
C	Compound (open)
D	Compression
E	Greenstick
F	Impacted
G	Intra-articular
H	Oblique
I	Spiral
J	Transverse

From the list above, select the single most likely type of fracture sustained in each of the following clinical scenarios. The items may be used once, more than once or not at all.

1 The casualty officer calls you to refer a 'volar Barton's' fracture in an elderly woman, who fell onto her outstretched hand.

2 A young boy gets his ankle caught while running across a cattle grid, stumbles and falls to the floor applying an external rotation to his leg. He presents to casualty with a visibly deformed femur.

3 An elderly woman slips on the floor of her kitchen and lands on her back. She is unable to weight bear and is brought to casualty via ambulance. On examination, she has severe restriction of all movements of her right hip and is unable to straight leg raise. Despite her X-ray showing a minimally displaced fracture of her neck of femur she does **not** have a shortened or externally rotated leg.

162 CLASSIFICATION OF FRACTURES

1** **G – Intra-articular**
Barton described an intra-articular fracture of the distal radius. Strictly, the original description related to fracture of the anterior portion of the radius. However, the term is commonly used for *all* intra-articular distal radius fractures.

2 **I – Spiral**

3 **F – Impacted**
This is Garden 1 fracture and is impacted.

- See ERN MRCS Book 2, Chapter 2, section 7.1.

- Classification of fractures involves the description of:

  - fracture pattern
  - position
  - angulation
  - displacement
  - soft tissue disruption.

- (Eponymous) classification systems (eg Gartland, Salter–Harris etc) merely incorporate such parameters.

- An adequate description of any fracture should incorporate **all** such information. For example: a closed, transverse, supracondylar fracture, which is off ended and is angulated by 30° (a Gartland 3 fracture).

- The fracture type may give an idea of the mechanism of injury, energy of the injury, damage to soft tissue structures and the likely best treatment.

163 THEME: PRINCIPLES OF FRACTURE MANAGEMENT

A	Broad arm sling
B	Collar and cuff
C	Dynamic plate and screw
D	External fixation/Ilizarov frame
E	Intramedullary fixation
F	Joint replacement (hemi/total arthroplasty)
G	Plaster of Paris immobilisation
H	Plate and screws
I	Screw fixation
J	Traction

From the list above select the single most appropriate treatment option for the following fractures. The items may be used once, more than once or not at all.

☐ 1 A 38-year-old motorcyclist is involved in a road traffic accident and presents to A&E with a haemarthrosis of his right knee. X-rays show a minimally displaced fracture of his lateral femoral condyle.

☐ 2 A 42-year-old builder falls from a second story scaffold onto soft ground. He is brought to A&E with a severely deformed lower leg and evidence of a (extra-articular) pilon fracture.

☐ 3 A 23-year-old girl falls awkwardly, while wearing high heels, following the consumption of copious quantities of alcohol. She presents the following morning having woken and been unable to weight bear. On examination she has a significantly swollen ankle with restriction of movement. X-ray reveals a bimalleolar fracture with talar tilt.

☐ A 78-year-old osteoporotic woman falls onto her outstretched arm while getting out of a car. She attends A&E with a painful swollen shoulder with a global reduction in movements. Radiographs reveal a fracture of the surgical neck of the humerus angulated by 30° and off-ended by 80%.

1**   **C – Dynamic plate and screw**
A dynamic compression screw is placed at 90° across the femoral condyles.

2   **D – External fixation Ilizarov frame**
A pilon fracture describes a badly comminuted distal tibia and fibula fracture.

3   **H – Plate and screws**

4   **B – Collar and cuff**

- See ERN MRCS Book 2, Chapter 2, section 7.1.

- Consideration of the fracture site, dynamics and mechanism of injury will allow selection of the optimum method of management. In clinical practice, there are frequently several options available.

- A dynamic compression screw is similar to a dynamic hip screw but has an angle of fixation of 90°. It is the fixation of choice for femoral condylar fractures, as it obviates the need for massive joint replacement (buttress plating would also be acceptable not offered as an option here).

- External fixation is appropriate in badly comminuted fractures.

- Plate and screw fixation is widely accepted as treatment of choice for ankle fractures with disruption to the mortice (indicated here by talar tilt).

- A collar and cuff provides adequate traction (via gravity) to treat all two-part and undisplaced three-part humeral head fractures.

164 THEME: COMPLICATIONS OF FRACTURES 1

A   Arthritis
B   Avascular necrosis
C   Compartment syndrome
D   Delayed union
E   Epiphyseal injury
F   Fat embolism
G   Infection
H   Malunion
I   Myositis ossificans
J   Neurological injury
K   Non-union
L   Reflex sympathetic dystrophy
M   Tendon injury
N   Vascular injury
O   Volkmann's ischaemic contracture

From the list above pick the single most likely complication of the fractures described in each of the following clinical scenarios. The items may be used once, more than once or not at all.

1   A 78-year-old woman suffers a Colles-type distal radius fracture, which is successfully manipulated and immobilised in a cast. Six weeks later when the cast is removed the patient is still complaining of shooting 'electric-type' pains across the dorsum of her hand that do not respond to simple analgesics. Radiographic evaluation shows a fracture that has healed well.

2   A 23-year-old man re-presents to the fracture clinic 3 months following a minimally displaced scaphoid wrist fracture, which was managed in a scaphoid cast. He complains of ongoing stiffness and pain in the joint. X-rays are normal.

3   A 35-year-old man sustains closed tibia and fibula shaft fractures in a road traffic accident. As it is late at night, the decision is made to leave the definitive management of this injury until the morning and skin traction is applied. You are called to the ward 4 hours later as the patient is now complaining of severe pain, which is disproportionate to the injury and not relieved by morphine. Sensation and pulses are intact.

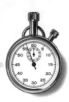
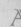

164 COMPLICATIONS OF FRACTURES 1

1**   **L – Reflex sympathetic dystrophy**
Synonyms: Sudeck's atrophy; complex regional pain syndrome.

2   **B – Avascular necrosis**

3   **C – Compartment syndrome**

- See ERN MRCS Book 2, Chapter 2, section 7.13.

- Favourite complications tested in examinations include fat embolism, complex regional pain syndromes, avascular necrosis, non-union/delayed union and compartment syndrome

- Complex regional pain syndrome is a poorly understood phenomenon presenting with severe post-traumatic pain associated with disturbances to the sympathetic nerve supply.

- Avascular necrosis following trauma is classically associated with bones with a retrograde blood supply, ie **scaphoid, neck of femur, lunate, talus**. It classically presents with ongoing pain and stiffness. X-rays may show no early changes but later show involution and distortion of the bone shape.

- Compartment syndrome must be suspected in any patient with disproportionate pain following a long bone fracture. Measurement of compartment pressures may aid diagnosis but it is **primarily** a clinical diagnosis. Fasciotomy must not be delayed.

165 THEME: COMPLICATIONS OF FRACTURES 2

A   Arthritis
B   Avascular necrosis
C   Compartment syndrome
D   Cross union
E   Delayed union
F   Epiphyseal injury
G   Fat embolism
H   Infection
I   Malunion
P   Myositis ossificans
J   Neurological injury
K   Non-union
L   Reflex sympathetic dystrophy
M   Tendon injury
N   Vascular injury
O   Volkmann's ischaemic contracture

From the list above pick the single most likely complication of the fractures described in each of the following clinical scenarios. The items may be used once, more than once or not at all.

1   A 9-year-old boy sustains a fracture of his distal radius in a 'bouncy castle'. This is reduced and held with three percutaneous K-wires. Check X-rays taken at the time revealed good reduction and fixation. However, he re-presents 1 year later complaining that one arm is shorter than the other.

2   A 29-year-old roofer falls from the second floor, sustaining nasty fractures of his radius and ulna. The ulna is plated but the radius is minimally displaced and managed in a cast. During the following weeks there is a delay in the union of the fracture, which eventually heals. You review him in fracture clinic and he now complains of pain and stiffness. Examination reveals absent pronation.

3   A 37-year-old jockey is thrown from his horse and sustains bilateral femoral shaft fractures. He undergoes bilateral nailing that evening, and you are called to see him later that night. He is tachycardic, short of breath and is complaining of mild chest tightness.

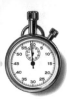

165 COMPLICATIONS OF FRACTURES 2

1   F – Epiphyseal injury

2**   D – Cross union

3   G – Fat embolus

- See ERN MRCS Book 2, Chapter 2, section 7.13.

- Damage to the growth plate may present late with limb length discrepancy.

- Cross union is a rare condition occurring in the distal radius and ulna. It is seen in delayed or slow healing fractures.

- Fat embolus is a rare but potentially fatal condition classically seen after long bone fractures and burns. The pathogenesis remains unclear, although it is likely to be due to either the spillage of marrow into the systemic circulation or the activities of lipase released into the circulation as part of systemic inflammatory response syndrome.

166 THEME: EPONYMOUS UPPER LIMB INJURIES

A	Barton's (dorsal) fracture
B	Barton's (volar) fracture
C	Bennett's fracture
D	Colles' fracture
E	Galeazzi's fracture
F	Rolando's fracture
G	Smith's fracture
H	Stener–Lesion fracture

From the list above select the single most likely diagnosis for the following clinical scenarios. The items may be used once, more than once or not at all.

1　A 79-year-old woman with osteoporosis trips and falls over a rug in her kitchen. She lands on her outstretched hand and presents to casualty with a 'dinner fork' deformity.

2　A young man presents to A&E having fallen from a trampoline onto his outstretched hand. He has an obvious deformity of the forearm with a palpable ulna head. X-rays reveal a mid-shaft radius fracture.

3　You are shown an X-ray by the A&E officer who asks whether he may 'pull' this Colles' fracture. You note that there is intra-articular extension of this dorsally angulated and impacted fracture and advise **against** his proposed course of action.

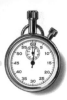

166 EPONYMOUS UPPER LIMB INJURIES

1   D – Colles' fracture
2   E – Galeazzi's fracture
3   A – Barton's (dorsal) fracture

- See ERN MRCS Book 2, Chapter 2, sections 7.2–7.5.

- Common eponymous injuries of the upper limb:

  - Colles' fracture: distal radius fracture. Clinically, a dinner fork deformity is seen. The radius is impacted, dorsally angulated and radially deviated.
  - Barton's fracture: an intra-articular distal radius fracture. Better described by Frykman.
  - Bennett's fracture: an intra-articular fracture dislocation of the base of the thumb, where only the volar ulna fragment is held in place.
  - Galeazzi's fracture: a mid-shaft radius fracture with concomitant dislocation of the distal radius–ulna junction.
  - Monteggia fracture: a mid-shaft ulna fracture with a radial head dislocation.
  - Smith's fracture: similar to a Colles' fracture but with **volar** angulation. Contrary to popular belief, this fracture is **not** caused by falling onto a flexed wrist.
  - Rolando's fracture: a three-part fracture of the base of the thumb metacarpal.

167 THEME: UPPER LIMB PERIPHERAL NERVE INJURIES

A   Axillary nerve
B   Erb's palsy
C   Median nerve
D   Musculocutaneous nerve
E   Radial nerve
F   Ulnar nerve – proximal
G   Ulnar nerve – distal

From the list above, select the single most likely nerve injury described in each of the following clinical scenarios. The items may be used once, more than once or not at all.

1   A 45-year-old rugby player presents to A&E after a night out with the team. He tells you his wife made him sleep on the sofa last night. When he awoke this morning he is unable to extend his wrist. He has a small sensory deficit over the base of the thumb.

2   A 19-year-old girl punches through a plate glass window in a rage. Although she does not suffer any vascular injury, she presents with a claw deformity of the hand and loss of sensation over the ulnar one and half digits.

3   A 17-year-old boy with chronic, poorly controlled epilepsy previously attended A&E following a fit. He was noted to have a dislocated shoulder, which was reduced using longitudinal traction. On review in orthopaedic clinic, he has evidence of weakness of elbow flexion and supination. Documented examination following the initial reduction showed no sensory deficit over the 'axillary badge' area.

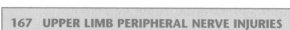

1   E – Radial nerve

2   G – Ulnar nerve – distal

3**   D – Musculocutaneous nerve

- See ERN MRCS Book 2, Chapter 2, section 3.17.

- The patient has suffered an anterior shoulder dislocation (common during fits). Although he does not present with axillary nerve palsy, he have evidence of musculocutaneous nerve palsy (biceps), which may also complicate anterior shoulder dislocation.

- The table gives a summary of upper limb peripheral nerve injuries:

Nerve	Roots	Innervation	Features with palsy
Axillary	C5/6	Deltoid, teres minor. Sensation to axillary badge	Sensory loss and weak abduction of arm
Median	C6–T1	'LOAF' Flexor carpi radialis, flexor digitalis profundus, pronator teres. Sensation to radial three and a half digits	Wasting of thenar eminence. Sensory loss radial three and a half digits
Musculocutaneous	C5/6	Biceps, brachialis, coracobrachialis	Weakness in arm flexion. Sensory deficit variable or absent
Ulnar	C8/T1	Flexor carpi ulnaris, flexor digitalis profundus. Medial two lumbricales. Sensation to ulnar one and a half digits. Interosseus muscles, adductor pollicis	High – loss of sensation to ulnar one and a half digits, weakness in abduction of fingers. *No claw hand* (ulnar paradox). Low – as above, but with claw hand
Radial	C6,7,8	Triceps, supinator, and wrist extensors.	Wrist drop (*Saturday night palsy*)

168 THEME: MANAGEMENT OF PELVIC FRACTURES

A   Conservative treatment
B   External fixation of the pelvis
C   Stabilisation through binding of the pelvis
D   Stabilisation through binding of the pelvis and then external fixation

From the list above, select the single most appropriate treatment in the first 8 hours following pelvic injury for the following clinical scenarios. In all cases adequate ongoing resuscitation is assumed. The items may be used once, more than once or not at all.

☐ 1 A 97-year-old woman presents to A&E following a fall. Although she is alert and orientated, she is unable to weight bear due to pain in her hip. Radiological investigation reveals fractures of the right superior and inferior pubic rami.

☐ 2 You attend a trauma call, involving a 23-year-old woman, who has been hit on her side by a train. She is cardiovascularly unstable. There are no clinical or radiological signs of significant chest or abdominal injury. Trauma radiographs reveal disruption of the pubic symphysis and sacroiliac joints.

☐ 3 A 49-year-old builder attends A&E after some heavy machinery fell on him. Although alert and orientated, he is persistently tachycardic but has no evidence of occult haemorrhage. His trauma radiographs demonstrate a pelvic fracture involving the pubic rami and iliac wing.

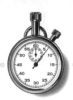

168 MANAGEMENT OF PELVIC FRACTURES

1   **A – Conservative treatment**
     This is a stable injury.

2** **D – Stabilisation through binding of the pelvis and then external fixation.**
     An open book injury is described.

3   **C – Stabilisation through binding of the pelvis**
     A lateral compression (LC) 2 injury is described

•   See ERN MRCS Book 2, Chapter 2, section 7.11 and pelvic fractures (www.bonedoctors.co.uk/pelvis/young.htm).

•   Pelvic injuries are potentially life threatening due to the opportunity for massive haemorrhage into the large space within the pelvis.

•   Expansion of the pelvic volume results in tearing of the venous plexuses surrounding the sacrum and lumbar spine.

•   In addition to aggressive resuscitation in accordance with ATLS principles, treatment of volume expanding pelvic fractures is to reduce the volume. It is rare that the pelvis needs to be packed, but this can be considered in extreme cases.

•   External fixation is indicated in all severely unstable pelvic injuries but binding of the pelvis and bed rest may suffice in less severe injuries.

•   Acetabular fractures **never** require binding or external fixation to the pelvis.

169 THEME: HIP FRACTURES

A   Bed rest
B   Conservative treatment
C   Dynamic hip screw
D   Femoral nail
E   Hemiarthroplasty
F   Proximal femoral recon nail
G   Total hip replacement
H   Traction

From the list above, select the single most appropriate method of fixation of the fractures described in the following clinical scenarios. The items may be used once, more than once or not at all.

☐   1   A 38-year-old woman attends A&E following a fall from her horse. She is unable to weight bear due to hip pain. AP and lateral X-rays confirm the clinical suspicion of a subcapital fracture dislocation of the right femoral neck.

☐   2   A 62-year-old asthmatic man presents following low energy fall with pain in his right leg. Examination reveals severely restricted movements and a shortened and externally rotated leg. X-rays demonstrate a displaced femoral neck fracture on a background of osteopenia.

☐   3   A 78-year-old arthritic woman slips awkwardly on the ice while carrying her shopping. She is transferred to hospital via ambulance and is found to have a reverse, oblique subtrochanteric proximal femoral fracture.

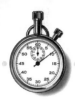

1**   C – Dynamic hip screw

2   G – Total hip replacement
Although the patient could have a hemiarthroplasty, a young high-demand user should have a cemented total arthroplasty, especially in the presence of osteopenia.

3   F – Proximal femoral recon nail

- See ERN MRCS Book 2, Chapter 2, section 7.6.

- Proximal femoral fractures in young patients (< 40 years) are an orthopaedic emergency. The patient must be treated with internal fixation (dynamic hip screw or recon nail) within 4 hours of injury to minimise the risk of avascular necrosis.

- Intracapsular fractures (subcapital and intracapsular) should be treated with total or hemiarthroplasty, as the retrograde blood supply is likely to be compromised.

- Intertrochanteric fractures should be treated with intramedullary fixation (either dynamic hip screw or recon nail). Reverse oblique fractures should be treated with recon nailing.

- Subtrochanteric fractures should be treated with intramedullary fixation.

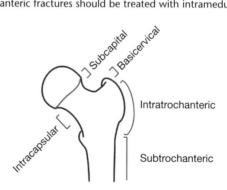

Reproduced from: http://www.bonedoctors.co.uk (c) 2006 *Ben Ollivere*, with kind permission.

170 THEME: LOWER LIMB FRACTURES

A	Displaced fracture manageable in a cast
B	Displaced fracture requiring no treatment
C	Displaced fracture requiring operative fixation
D	Displaced fracture requiring traction
E	Undisplaced fracture manageable in a cast
F	Undisplaced fracture requiring no treatment
G	Undisplaced fracture requiring operative fixation
H	Undisplaced fracture requiring traction

From the list above, select the single most appropriate treatment for each of the following clinical scenarios. The items may be used once, more than once or not at all.

1 A 24-year-old semiprofessional hurdler sustains an injury following a difficult landing during training. He attends A&E ankle pain and a limp. Although he is able to weight bear, X-rays reveal a minimally displaced Weber B ankle fracture with 3 mm of talar shift.

2 A 38-year-old cricketer presents with a painful swollen patella following a direct blow from a cricket ball. He is able to straight leg raise with difficulty. X-ray examination shows a mildly displaced patella fracture.

3 A 17-year-old girl falls from her horse and is dragged several feet as her foot became stuck in the stirrup. She presents with a swollen deformed foot that is acutely tender over the second metatarsal head.

171 THEME: LOWER LIMB NERVE INJURIES

A	Common peroneal nerve	E	Sciatic nerve
B	Diabetic neuropathy	F	Sural nerve injury
C	Femoral nerve	G	Systemic demyelination
D	Reflex sympathetic dystrophy		

From the list above, select the single most likely diagnosis for each of the following clinical scenarios. The items may be used once, more than once or not at all.

1 A 23-year-old man is reviewed in orthopaedic clinic 28 days after undergoing plate fixation of a fractured os calcis. He complains of some slight stiffness at the subtalar joint and also of numbness on the lateral aspect of his foot and ankle.

You are called by the physiotherapist to review a 67-year-old woman who is 24 hours post total knee replacement. She is concerned as the patient appears to have developed unilateral 'foot drop'.

3 An 87-year-old man presents to the orthopaedic clinic with difficulty walking. He gives a history of a recent increase in shoe size. On examination, he has a pes planus foot. Neurological examination reveals circumferential sensory loss affecting the distal lower leg and foot.

170 LOWER LIMB FRACTURES

1   **G – Undisplaced fracture requiring operative fixation**

2   **A – Displaced fracture manageable in a cast**

3**   **C – Displaced fracture requiring operative fixation**

- See ERN MRCS Book 2, Chapter 2, section 7.8.

- All ankle fractures are potentially intra-articular and meticulous reduction is required. Low demand users or patients with undisplaced fractures may be managed in a cast. Talar shift is an indication for fixation in this case, as is the high demand nature of the user.

- Patella fractures are manageable in a cast if the extensor mechanism is intact. Complex fractures or those with disruption to the extensors may require tension band wiring.

- Lisfranc's injury was originally described in cavalry officers during the Crimean war. This is a serious 'forefoot on mid-foot' fracture dislocation and requires urgent operative management.

171 LOWER LIMB NERVE INJURIES

1**   **F – Sural nerve palsy**

2   **A – Common peroneal nerve**

3   **B – Diabetic neuropathy**

- See ERN MRCS Book 2, Chapter 2, section 2.14.

- The sural nerve has no motor function, and is entirely sensory and autonomic in function.

- The common peroneal nerve is at risk during knee replacement surgery. It is most often damaged by a lateral retractor as it spirals round the fibula.

- The most common neurological condition of the lower limb is diabetic neuropathy, which presents with Charcot's joints and stocking distribution sensory loss.

172 THEME: MANAGEMENT OF SOFT TISSUE INJURIES

A Wound wash out and closure
B Wound wash out and leave open
C Wound wash out, debridement and closure
D Wound wash out, debridement and leave open

From the list above, select the single most appropriate management of the soft tissue injuries described in each of the following clinical scenarios. The items may be used once, more than once or not at all.

1 A 17-year-old boy presents with a large laceration to his forearm following a dog bite. The wound does not appear to be grossly contaminated.

2 A 47-year-old motorcyclist presents with a large open fracture to his left tibia and fibula. The wound is contaminated with grit and debris.

3 A 15-year-old girl is taken to hospital following spillage of concentrated sulphuric acid on her leg during a chemistry lesson. The child has a 3.5 × 7 cm cavity on the anterior aspect of her thigh, which is 1 cm deep.

173 THEME: COMMON DISORDERS OF THE FOOT

A Hallux valgus
B Hammer toe
C March fracture
D Morton's neuroma
E Pes planus
F Plantar fasciitis
G Tibialis posterior insufficiency

From the list above, select the single most likely diagnosis for each of the following clinical scenarios. The items may be used once, more than once or not at all.

1 A 35-year-old schoolteacher complains of significant pain over the plantar aspect of her foot. It is particularly noticeable when standing from her desk at work. She complains of 'crippling pain' and she finds it difficult to walk. The pain 'eases off' once she becomes mobile. On examination, she is tender over the antero-inferior aspect of the calcaneum. Radiographs show a calcaneal spur.

2 A 31-year-old marathon runner presents to casualty with pain across his entire foot. There is no visible swelling, although he is mildly tender over several of the metatarsals. Radiographs exclude the presence of any fractures but you notice several areas of cortical thickening affecting the metatarsals.

3 A 53-year-old woman presents to the orthopaedic clinic complaining of pain across the plantar aspect of her foot. She can only wear 'extra wide' shoes. Examination reveals a widened forefoot with significant callus formation over the first and second metatarsal heads, along with deformity of the great toe.

---

172 MANAGEMENT OF SOFT TISSUE INJURIES

1** D – Wound wash out, debridement and leave open

2   D – Wound wash out, debridement and leave open

3   D – Wound wash out, debridement and leave open

- See ERN MRCS Book 1, Chapter 1, section 2.1; ERN MRCS Book 2, Chapter 2, section 5.8; and the British Orthopaedic Association, publications. Guidelines on management of open fractures and significant soft tissue injuries.

- All (potentially) contaminated soft tissue injuries must be explored, washed out and debrided to healthy tissue. The wound should be lightly packed and dressed and the patient taken for a second look in 24 hours. Closure may be contemplated 24 hours later (delayed primary closure).

- Antibiotics and tetanus should be given as appropriate.

---

173 COMMON DISORDERS OF THE FOOT

1** F – Plantar fasciitis

2   C – March fracture

3   A – Hallux valgus

- See ERN MRCS Book 2, Chapter 2, section 2.15.

- Plantar fasciitis is a common condition of mixed aetiology, which is characterised by pain over the plantar aspect of the foot, typically when rising from standing. Calcaneal bone spurs are said to be pathological. Treatment with steroid injections may be of some help.

- March fractures present in individuals who undergo repeated low-grade trauma. Although no specific cortical breach is seen, multiple microfractures result in pain. The classic radiological finding is of cortical thickening from callus formation.

- Hallux valgus is a lateral subluxation of the metatarsalphalangeal (MTP) joint of the great toe – commonly known as a 'bunion'. It may be treated by a variety of osteotomies or by fusion of the joint.

- Morton's neuroma is a small painful neuroma seen classically between the third and fourth toes. Diagnosis may be confirmed on MRI scan. Surgical excision will resolve symptoms.

174 THEME: MONOARTHRITIS

A Gout
B Osteoarthritis
C Pseudogout
D Psoriatic arthritis
E Reactive synovitis
F Rheumatoid arthritis
G Septic arthritis

From the list above, select the most likely diagnosis for each of the following clinical scenarios. The items may be used once, more than once or not at all.

1 A 65-year-old woman presents to clinic with increasing pain and stiffness in her right leg. Specifically, she reports anterior knee pain and associated swelling. She has difficulty climbing stairs and says that the pain is relieved by rest.

2 A 67-year-old man presents to casualty 3 weeks following anterior cruciate ligament repair with an acutely painful hot and swollen knee. He is able to weight bear but with some difficulty. Examination reveals an acutely tender, hot swollen joint. The knee is held in 30° of flexion and his range of movement is limited from 25° to 45°.

3 A 43-year-old woman presents with an acute onset of a hot, swollen, painful wrist. She has no history of trauma. Examination confirms restriction of all movements. Her WCC is 10^9/L and her C-reactive protein level is 47. Radiographs reveal radio-opaque lines within the joint space itself.

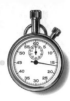

174 MONOARTHRITIS

1   **B – Osteoarthritis**

2   **G – Septic arthritis**

3**   **C – Pseudogout**
The lines represent chondral calcification.

- See ERN MRCS Book 2, Chapter 2, sections 1.5, 1.6 and 5.2.

- For a summary of arthropathies see table in Answer 175.

175 THEME: POLYARTHRITIS

A	Ankylosing spondylitis
B	Gout
C	Osteoarthritis
D	Pseudogout
E	Psoriatic arthritis
F	Reactive synovitis
G	Rheumatoid arthritis
H	Septic arthritis

From the list above, select the most likely diagnosis for each of the following clinical scenarios. The items may be used once, more than once or not at all.

☐ 1 You are asked to see an anxious 24-year-old woman in A&E. During the past few days, she has developed pain and swelling affecting the interphalangeal (IP) joints of her right hand. On examination, there is tenderness and 'boggy' swelling over the IP joints of the hand. The left hand is also affected but to a much lesser extent. There is a silvery patch of skin over her elbow but nothing else of note.

☐ 2 A mother brings her 5-year-old son to the A&E department. He has been complaining pains in his legs and arms for the last 16 hours. He is able to mobilise but has painful, restricted movements in the hips and knees. Radiographs are unremarkable. On direct questioning, his mother tells you that he has just recovered from a coryzal illness.

☐ 3 A 47-year-old car mechanic is referred to clinic with symmetrical pain in both hips and his lower back. Examination is unremarkable. X-ray of the lumbar spine reveals syndesmophytes and loss of lordosis.

175 POLYARTHRITIS

1   **E – Psoriatic arthritis**
2   **F – Reactive synovitis**
3   **A – Ankylosing spondylitis**
•   See ERN MRCS Book 2, Chapter 2, sections 1.5, 1.6 and 5.2.
•   The table summarises monoarthropathies/polyarthropathies:

Arthropathy	Epidemiology	Joints	Aetiology	Presentation
Inflammatory	Inflammatory bowel disease	Poly/sacroiliac joints	Uncertain, possibly immune complex	Patients with established inflammatory bowel disease. Polyarthritis may be first presenting symptom
	Rheumatoid	Polyarthritis Symmetrical Metacarpophalangeal joints	Autoimmune Rh factor driven	Polyarthritis commonly affecting the distal interphalangeal joints in hands. Systemic symptoms sometimes present. Classically present in young women
	Psoriatic arthritis	Asymmetrical poly, interphalangeal joints	Autoimmune	In association with cutaneous psoriasis
	Ankylosing spondylitis	Spine/hips	Chronic inflammation	Pain and stiffness of back/hips. Syndesmophytes and bamboo spine (gives rise to 'question mark' posture)
Crystals	Gout	Monoarthritis. metatarsophalangeal (MTP)/knee/wrist	Urate crystal deposition	Acute onset monoarthritis classically in the MTP joint. Associated tophi formation. Birefringent crystals
	Pseudogout	Monoarthritis. MTP/knee/wrist	Calcium phosphate crystal deposition	Similar to gout, but with chondrocalcinosis
Degenerative	Osteoarthritis	Mono/poly Major joints first and spine Asymmetrical	Exact aetiology unknown Erosive arthritis	Classically seen in the sixth/seventh decade Large joints affected first. Cartilage loss and loss of joint space earliest signs Pain and stiffness in the morning
	Post-traumatic	Mono	Intra-articular fracture or malunited fracture causing uneven wear	Several years post injury. Early-onset osteoarthritis affecting joint with previous fracture
Infective/ reactive	Septic arthritis	Mono	Septic infection of bone space	Acutely swollen, tender joint Systemic upset Raised WCC
	Reactive synovitis	Poly	Post viral	Multiple joints Stiffness, aching and pain

176 THEME: INFECTIONS OF BONE

A	Acute haematogenous osteomyelitis
B	Acute post-traumatic/post-operative osteomyelitis
C	Acute suppurative arthritis
D	Chronic osteomyelitis
E	Tuberculous arthritis
F	Reactive synovitis
G	No infection – other pathology

From the list above, select the most likely diagnosis for each of the following clinical scenarios. The items may be used once, more than once or not at all.

1 A 59-year-old Indian woman presents with a 3-year history of right knee pain. She has been previously diagnosed with arthritis by her GP. On examination, the right knee is swollen joint with synovial thickening. There is evidence of wasting of the ipsilateral quadriceps. Radiographs reveal a significant loss of joint space in the presence of osteoporotic change.

2 You are asked to review a patient on ICU who is requiring non-invasive ventilation and inotropic support following an intra-operative myocardial infarction during an elective AAA repair. The ICU staff have noticed a swollen, erythematous left elbow. On examination, the joint is warm and there is global restriction of range of movements.

3 A patient attends the orthopaedic clinic 1 year following fixation of a Weber A ankle fracture. She still has a plate and screws medially and two cancellous screws laterally. She has experienced pain in the ankle since the time of the injury but has been reassured that this is probably related to the trauma itself. On examination, there is an area of induration and a discharging sinus over the site of the plate medially.

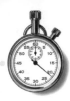

176 INFECTIONS OF BONE

1**   **E – Tuberculous arthritis**
Classical presentation described.

2   **A – Acute haematogenous osteomyelitis**
Patient will have multiple arterial/venous/endoluminal lines.

3   **D – Chronic osteomyelitis**

- See ERN MRCS Book 2, Chapter 2, section 5.

- A diagnosis of tuberculous arthritis must be considered in all patients originating from areas of the world where tuberculosis is prevalent.

- The causative organism of bone infections may, as a general rule, be considered thus:

  - origin from tuberculosis endemic regions = tuberculosis
  - other patients: age < 4 years = *Haemophilus influenzae* or > 4 years = *Staphylococcus aureus*.

- Acute haematogenous osteomyelitis is often seen in the immunocompromised or acutely unwell with indwelling venous lines.

177 THEME: BACK PAIN

A	Anterior cord syndrome
B	Brown–Sequard syndrome
C	Central cord syndrome
D	Disc prolapse
E	Lateral cord syndrome
F	Mechanical back pain
G	Pott's disease
H	Spinal stenosis
I	Spondylolisthesis

From the list above, select the most likely diagnosis for each of the following clinical scenarios. The items may be used once, more than once or not at all.

1 A 57-year-old man presents to casualty after falling 1.8 metres (6 feet) from a ladder. Although his radiographs are unremarkable, he presents with weakness in both arms. The A&E SHO is puzzled when making the referral as there are no neurological signs affecting the lower limb and perianal sensation is intact.

2 A 17-year-old gymnast attends A&E with back pain following a competition. Her GP has noted astutely that she has a distended abdomen and refers her to the general surgical team with a working diagnosis of visceral haemorrhage. However, she is haemodynamically stable and her haemoglobin concentration is 132 g/l (13.2 g/dl) and an FAST scan of the abdomen is unremarkable.

3 You are asked to see a 67-year-old arteriopathic man in the outpatient clinic by your vascular colleagues. He was initially referred to them with a history of claudication. The pain is induced by exercise, particularly walking *downhill* rather than uphill, and is relieved by rest. However, angiogram has excluded the presence of significant peripheral occlusive arterial disease.

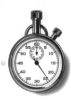

177 BACK PAIN

1   **C – Central cord syndrome**

2**   **I – Spondylolisthesis**
A distended abdomen is commonly seen due to anterior slip.

3   **H – Spinal stenosis**
This leads to *spinal* claudication.

- See ERN MRCS Book 2, Chapter 6, section 2.5.

- Cord compression must **always** be excluded in patients presenting with back pain.

- Mechanical pain – transient backache, often following muscular activity. Responds to rest and graded exercise.

- Anterior cord syndrome – complete paralysis, but sparing of the dorsal columns (deep pressure and proprioception) to the lower limbs

- Central cord syndrome – disproportionately greater motor impairment in upper compared to lower limbs. Sensory loss is variable, although sacral sensation is usually present.

- Brown–Sequard syndrome – usually due to penetrating thoracic injuries. Cord hemisection results in ipsilateral motor dysfunction and contralateral loss of pain and temperature sensation.

- Spinal stenosis – aching numbness and paraesthesia, particularly after standing upright. Relieved by sitting or squatting and may often be asymmetrical. Due to degenerate changes narrowing of the spinal canal.

- Spondylolisthesis – subluxation (usually of bone L4 on L5). Classically seen in adolescent children undergoing hyperflexion of the spine, eg in gymnastics.

- Disc prolapse – associated with cord or nerve root signs. Sudden-onset backache with shooting sciatic pain ± paraesthesia and absent reflexes is pathognomonic. Loss of rectal tone and altered perianal sensation suggests significant cord compromise.

178 THEME: BONE AND SOFT TISSUE TUMOURS

A	Bone cyst
B	Chondrosarcoma
C	Giant cell tumour
D	Metastatic bone tumour
E	Multiple myeloma
F	Osteochondroma
G	Osteoidosteoma
H	Osteosarcoma

From the list above, select the most likely diagnosis for each of the following clinical scenarios. The items may be used once, more than once or not at all.

☐ 1 A 15-year-old girl presents with a hard lump on the medial aspect of her proximal tibia, overlying the epiphysial plate. The patient has normal function in her knee, although she does experience some pain in the lump.

☐ 2 A 32-year-old clergyman presents with some pain and swelling in his knee. He was seen by his GP, who made a diagnosis of infra-patella bursitis. When the problem failed to resolve the GP arranged an X-ray, which reveals an 8-cm rarefied asymmetrical area abutting the subchondral bone of the tibia.

☐ 3 A 49-year-old man presents to fracture clinic with a fractured humeral neck. He describes a 3-month history of generalised pain in his shoulder, backache, malaise and weakness. X-rays demonstrate osteoporotic-looking bone with an osteolytic lesion evident. Laboratory tests are unremarkable other than an ESR of 55 mm/h.

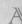

178 BONE AND SOFT TISSUE TUMOURS

1**   F – Osteochondroma

2**   C – Giant cell tumour

3   E – Multiple myeloma

- See ERN MRCS Book 2, Chapter 2, section 6.

- Osteochondromas are the commonest tumours of bone, and their commonest presentation is described. They may undergo malignant change.

- (Multinucleated) giant cell tumours occur in mature bone. One-third are benign, one-third locally invasive and one-third metastatic. The X-ray appearances described here are pathognomonic.

- Lassitude, pain, osteoporotic lesions and raised ESR = myeloma until proved otherwise.

179 THEME: PAEDIATRIC HIP DISORDERS

A   Congenital hip dysplasia
B   Irritable hip
C   Juvenile onset arthritis (Still's disease)
D   Perthes' disease (coax plana)
E   Septic arthritis
F   Slipped upper femoral epiphysis

From the list above, select the most likely diagnosis for each of the following clinical scenarios. The items may be used once, more than once or not at all.

☐   1   A 4-year-old boy presents with a painful limp. He has recently had a cough, which has now resolved. He looks well, and clinical examination reveals reduced movements at the right hip in all planes. His WCC is 10^9/L and his ESR is < 10 mm/h. Radiographic examination is normal.

☐   2   A 7-year-old boy presents for the second time to A&E. He reports chronic groin pain, and has a well-established limp. Examination reveals a stiff hip with pain at the extremes of movement. Abduction and internal rotation is severely limited.

☐   3   A 15-year-old boy presents with groin pain. Examination reveals an obese child with delayed sexual development. The pain came on acutely and radiates to the anterior thigh. Examination reveals a shortened and externally rotated leg.

1   B – Irritable hip

2**   D – Perthes' disease

3   F – Slipped upper femoral epiphysis

- See ERN MRCS Book 2, Chapter 2, section 4.1.

- A summary of paediatric hip disorders is provided in the table:

Age	Diagnosis	Symptoms	Investigations
Birth	Hip dysplasia	Asymmetrical creases and limited abduction	Ortolani's and Barlow's tests Ultrasound best investigation
0–5	Infections	Global restriction in movement. May be either reactive (ie irritable hip) or infective (ie septic arthritis)	Biochemistry, haematology and hip aspiration
5–10	Perthes' disease	Avascular necrosis of the femoral head. M:F = 4:1 Painful limp. Early stages: no X-ray changes	Not applicable
10–20	Slipped epiphysis	Extremely rare. Affects boys undergoing growth spurt. Ongoing history of groin pain in obese children age 10–15	X-ray shows widening of epiphysis
Adult	Osteoarthritis, rheumatoid arthritis, avascular necrosis	Depends on diagnosis	Radiological changes

180 THEME: METABOLIC BONE DISEASE

A   Acromegaly
B   Osteogenesis imperfecta
C   Osteoporosis
D   Osteomalacia
E   Paget's disease
F   Pott's disease
G   Primary hyperparathyroidism
H   Secondary hyperparathyroidism

From the list above, select the most likely diagnosis for each of the following clinical scenarios. The items may be used once, more than once or not at all.

1   A 45-year-old man presents to the outpatient clinic with generalised 'bone pain'. He has recently been diagnosed with diabetes mellitus. On direct questioning, he reports recent and surprising increase in his shoe size.

2   A 65-year-old woman is seen in orthopaedic outpatient clinic with anterior thigh and groin pain. Having made a provision diagnosis of osteoarthritis, you send her for X-rays, which reveal a 'flame-shaped' lytic lesion in her femoral shaft but no evidence of arthritic changes.

3   A 24-year-old Muslim woman experiences back and leg pain. Although normally active, she has to reduce her levels of activity and even finds walking upstairs troublesome.

181 THEME: SPINAL PATHOLOGY

A   Ankylosing spondylitis
B   Arthritic change
C   Metastatic tumour
D   Osteoporotic change
E   Pott's disease
F   Stable wedge fracture
G   Unstable wedge fracture

From the list above, select the most likely diagnosis for each of the following clinical scenarios. The items may be used once, more than once or not at all.

1   A 43-year-old man from the Indian subcontinent presents to clinic with a history of chronic lower back pain. Examination is unremarkable. Radiographs reveal wedging of the third lumbar vertebra and gibbus formation.

2   Following a high-energy road traffic accident, a 17-year-old drunk driver is blue-lighted to A&E. His only apparent injury is a two-column anterior wedge fracture of T7.

3   A 70-year-old heavy smoker is referred to the orthopaedic clinic with a progressively worsening kyphosis. He stands with difficulty and is hunched over. X-ray examination reveals osteopenic bone and multiple wedge fractures at all levels.

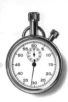

180 METABOLIC BONE DISEASE

1   A – Acromegaly

2** E – Paget's disease

3   D – Osteomalacia

- See ERN MRCS Book 2, Chapter 2, sections 1.7–1.10.

- Acromegaly is due to the excess production of growth hormone by pituitary tumours. Ten per cent present with diabetes, although glucose intolerance is more common. Thickening of the bone cortex and enlargement of the articular cartilage is characteristic.

- Paget's disease is often an incidental finding. Individuals may have isolated disease with no significant sequelae for many years.

- Osteomalacia (and rickets) is becoming less common as nutrition is improving. However, it may be seen in certain ethnic populations due to poor nutrition and/or avoidance of exposure to sunlight.

181 SPINAL PATHOLOGY

1   E – Pott's disease

2   F – Stable wedge fracture

3   D – Osteoporotic change

- See ERN MRCS Book 2, Chapter 2, sections 1.7 and 7.9 and Chapter 6, section 2.5.

- Pott's disease refers to tuberculosis of the spine. It should be suspected in patients from endemic regions of the world (eg Indian subcontinent).

- Osteoporosis may be primary or secondary. In this case, the clue is heavy smoking, leading to likely chronic obstructive pulmonary disease and steroid treatment.

- Classification of wedge fractures is based on the three columns (anterior, middle, posterior) as described by Denis. Greater than 50% loss of height is likely to be unstable. However, fractures of the thoracic spine are generally splinted by the rib cage.

UROLOGY

182 THEME: LOWER URINARY TRACT TRAUMA

A	CT scan of abdomen and pelvis
B	Furosemide 80 mg iv
C	Immediate laparotomy and exploration
D	Increase rate of iv infusion
E	Insert suprapubic catheter
F	Insert urethral catheter
G	Instil 50 ml of contrast into urethra followed by X-ray
H	Intravenous urogram (IVU)

From the list above, select the most appropriate next step in management for each of the following clinical scenarios. The items may be used once, more than once or not at all.

1 A 26-year-old man sustains an injury to the perineum by falling astride a beam. On examination, there is evidence of a butterfly perineal haematoma and there is blood at the external urethral meatus.

2 A 32-year-old man has sustained a road traffic accident. He is adequately resuscitated. Examination reveals fresh blood at the external urethral meatus. Radiographs reveal a fractured pubic ramus. Accordingly you request a retrograde urethrogram, which demonstrates a complete tear of the posterior urethra. His abdomen has become distended and uncomfortable. He has not passed urine since his arrival.

3 A 45-year-old man sustains a blow by the steering column to his lower abdomen during a road traffic accident. His primary and secondary surveys are complete. As he has not produced any urine and is found to have a high-riding prostate on digital rectal examination, you organise a urethrogram, which is essentially normal. However, bladder views are inadequate. Ultrasound scan of the pelvis reveals free fluid around the bladder.

182 LOWER URINARY TRACT TRAUMA

1   G – Instil 50 ml of contrast into urethra followed by X-ray

2   E – Insert suprapubic catheter

3**   H – IVU

- See ERN MRCS Book 1, Chapter 11, sections 3.4 and 3.5.

- Insertion of a urethral catheter should be **preceded** by a normal retrograde urethrogram when blood is present at the external urethral meatus.

- Repair of urethral injury is usually performed electively and thus urinary diversion via a suprapubic catheter is performed in the interim.

- Suspected bladder perforations can be investigated using retrograde (urethrogram) or antegrade (IVU) passage of contrast.

183 THEME: RENAL TRAUMA

A   Avulsion of the renal artery and vein
B   Extracapsular haematoma
C   Minor cortical laceration less than 1 cm deep without urinary leak
D   Parenchymal laceration extending into collecting system.
E   Parenchymal laceration more than 1 cm deep without urinary leak
F   'Shattered kidney' (multiple parenchymal lacerations)
G   Thrombosis of a renal artery
H   Thrombosis of a segmental artery without parenchymal laceration

From the list above, select the most likely pathology in each of the clinical scenarios described below. The items may be used once, more than once or not at all.

1   A 17-year-old youth is kicked in the right loin during a fight. On examination, he has severe bruising over the lower ribs and has evidence of microscopic haematuria. A CT scan of the abdomen and pelvis reveals a grade 1 renal injury.

2   A 30-year-old man is involved in a road traffic accident at 110 km/h (70 miles/h) that resulted in his vehicle leaving the road and hitting a tree. The ambulance crew have struggled to maintain a cardiac output during the 5-minute transfer. Despite resuscitation with 2 litres of crystalloid he has a faint pulse but no recordable blood pressure. Unfortunately, he arrests before definitive treatment can be instigated. Post-mortem examination confirms the diagnosis.

3   A 21-year-old man sustains a blow with a baseball bat to the left loin. He has evidence of macroscopic haematuria. A CT scan of the abdomen and pelvis confirms a grade 5 injury. Intravenous contrast is not taken up by a wedge-shaped area that occupies approximately one-fifth of the kidney.

183 RENAL TRAUMA

1   **B – Extracapsular haematoma**

2** **A – Avulsion of the renal artery and vein**
Prompt death following trauma (in this case within approximately 5–10 minutes of injury) usually implies major vessel injury.

3   **H – Thrombosis of a segmental artery without parenchymal laceration**

- See ERN MRCS Book 1, Chapter 11, section 3.2.

- 85% of renal trauma follows blunt injury.

- Initial management involves resuscitation in accordance with the principles of ATLS.

- CT scanning is the gold standard for the subsequent assessment of renal trauma.

- Miller and McAninch (1995) classified renal trauma into five grades.

  - I – contusion/haematoma
  - II – minor cortical laceration only
  - III – major cortical laceration extending into medulla only
  - IV – major laceration extending into collecting system
  - V – shattered kidney/pedicel avulsion leading to segmental devascularisation.

- Treatment is conservative (bed rest) unless there is evidence of:
  (i) haemodynamic instability; (ii) penetrating injury; (iii) persistent urinary extravasation; or (iv) retroperitoneal bleeding.

- Late complications include atrophic kidney or obstruction of the upper ureter due to fibrosis following urinoma/haematoma formation.

184 THEME: HAEMATURIA

A	Bladder diverticulum	F	Renal stone
B	Bladder stone	G	Transitional cell carcinoma
C	Endometriosis of the bladder		of the bladder
D	Prostate cancer	H	Urinary tract infection
E	Renal cell carcinoma		

From the list above, select the most likely diagnosis for each of the following clinical scenarios below. The items may be used once, more than once or not at all.

1 A 20-year-old sexually active woman complains of 'pink urine' and burning on micturition.

2 A 70-year-old man presents with frank haematuria and pain towards the end of micturition. He reports a sensation of incomplete bladder emptying and is able to urinate again after lying down for a while.

3 A 50-year-old woman presents to the outpatient clinic with frank haematuria. Several urine cultures taken by her GP have failed to reveal any growth. Her symptoms have persisted despite repeated courses of empirical antibiotic therapy.

185 THEME: PROSTATE CANCER

A	Cisplatin chemotherapy
B	Docetaxel chemotherapy
C	Luteinising hormone-releasing hormone (LHRH) analogue
D	LHRH antagonist
E	Radical radiotherapy
F	Radical retropubic prostatectomy
G	Tamsulosin
H	Transurethral resection of the prostate (TURP)

From the list above, select the most appropriate treatment for each of the following clinical scenarios below. The items may be used once, more than once or not at all.

1 A fit and well 50-year-old man is found to have a prostate-specific antigen (PSA) of 9.6 ng/ml at a 'routine check up' by his GP. Biopsy shows a Gleason 4+5 tumour in two cores. A CT scan confirms that the tumour is confined to the gland.

2 A 70-year-old man presents to his GP with acute on chronic backache. X-rays demonstrate sclerotic lesions in the lumbar vertebrae. Examination reveals no evidence of spinal cord compression. His PSA is 250 ng/ml.

3 A 70-year-old man has been on hormone suppression for advanced prostate cancer for some time. His PSA is now rising, despite several different hormone suppression regimens. He still enjoys a good quality of life and is keen to extend his life as much a possible, regardless of the possible side effects of treatment.

184 HAEMATURIA

1   H – Urinary tract infection

2**   B – Bladder stone

3   G – Transitional cell carcinoma of the bladder

- See ERN MRCS Book 1, Chapter 11, section 1.1.

- Urinary tract infection is the commonest cause of haematuria in young women. Investigation is only indicated if infections are persistent or recurrent despite adequate counselling regarding toilet habits and preventive strategies.

- Bladder stones can cause strangury (often with incomplete emptying) and haematuria.

- Smoking is associated with increased risk of transitional cell carcinoma of the bladder.

- Investigation of haematuria includes flexible cystoscopy and imaging of the upper tract.

185 PROSTATE CANCER

1   F – Radical retropubic prostatectomy

2**   C – LHRH analogue

3**   B – Docetaxel chemotherapy

- See ERN MRCS Book 1, Chapter 11, section 7.3.

- Fit, young patients with aggressive localised tumours are suitable for radical resection, usually via the retropubic approach.

- Prostate cancer spreads to bone causing sclerotic lesions, most commonly of the lumbar spine (90% metastases). These can cause cord compression.

- Hormone ablation shrinks tumours in almost all patients. Agents include antiandrogens and LHRH analogues, which decrease testosterone levels by reducing luteinising hormone production in the pituitary gland.

- Docetaxel (Taxotere) is the only chemotherapeutic agent to have a durable (modest) effect in hormone-resistant prostate cancer.

186 THEME: TESTICULAR TUMOURS

A   Choriocarcinoma
B   Epididymal carcinoma
C   Leydig cell tumours
D   Lymphoma
E   Non-seminomatous germ cell tumour
F   Seminoma
G   Sertoli cell tumour
H   Testicular microlithiasis

From the list above select the most likely diagnosis for each of the clinical scenarios below. The items may be used once, more than once or not at all.

1   A 25-year-old man presents with a testicular mass. His hCG and AFP levels are normal. Orchidectomy is performed and the histological examination reveals sheets of large, uniform cells. Follow up CT scanning demonstrates para-aortic lymphadenopathy, which subsequently responds well to radio-therapy.

2   A 27-year-old man has a positive urine pregnancy test and elevated serum AFP. He undergoes retroperitoneal lymph node dissection (RPLND), which is curative.

3   A 70-year-old man develops a scrotal swelling, which on investigation is found to be of a malignant nature.

1   F – Seminoma

2**   E – Non-seminomatous germ cell tumour

3   D – Lymphoma

- See ERN MRCS Book 1, Chapter 11, section 7.4.

- Seminomas:

  - 35% testis cancer
  - low AFP and hCG
  - radio sensitive and chemosensitive.

- Non-seminomatous germ cell tumours

  - 60% testis cancer
  - Include teratoma, embryonal cell carcinoma and mixed type
  - Removal of lymph nodes commonly curative (RPLND)
  - Chemotherapy may be used to treat recurrence.

- Non-germ cell tumours – rare, include Leydigs' cell and gonadoblastomas.

- Lymphoma is the commonest tumour in those over 55 years.

187 THEME: LOWER URINARY TRACT SYMPTOMS

A	Acute bacterial prostatitis
B	Benign prostatic enlargement
C	Chronic prostatitis
D	High-riding prostate
E	Normal prostate
F	Prostadynia
G	Prostate cancer
H	Prostatic calculus

From the list above, select the most likely diagnosis for each of the following clinical scenarios below. The items may be used once, more than once or not at all.

1 A 50-year-old man is referred to the outpatient clink with mixed lower urinary tract symptoms. On examination, there is a uniformly textured prostate with a volume of approximately 40 ml. His PSA is normal.

2 A 60-year-old man attends A&E with dysuria, malaise and generalised arthralgia. On digital examination of his rectum, the prostate gland is exquisitely tender.

3 A 55-year-old man is referred to the outpatient clinic with deteriorating lower urinary tract symptoms. On examination, he is found to have a craggy tender prostate. Urinalysis reveals 1+ of blood only.

187 LOWER URINARY TRACT SYMPTOMS

1**   **B – Benign prostatic enlargement**

2   **A – Acute bacterial prostatitis**

3   **G – Prostate cancer**

- See ERN MRCS Book 1, Chapter 11, sections 4.2 and 6.4.

- 'Lower urinary tract symptoms' (LUTs) refer to a collective term of symptoms that used to be referred to as 'prostatism'. However, causes other than merely prostatic pathology and pathophysiological mechanisms other than outlet obstruction may give rise to such symptoms. Bladder pathology (eg calculi/infection/tumours) may also result in similar symptoms.

- LUTs may be predominantly obstructive (hesitancy, poor stream, dribbling) or irritative (frequency, nocturia, urgency) and are assessed using the International Prostate Scoring System (IPSS).

- Benign prostatic enlargement is the same as benign prostatic hypertrophy (BPH). A volume of greater than 15 ml is considered moderate, and greater than 25 ml gross enlargement.

- PSA in combination with digital rectal examination is the best current screening test for prostate cancer. The specificity still seems to be too low to justify large-scale screening programmes.

188 THEME: ANTIBIOTICS

A	Amikacin 5 mg/kg iv three times daily
B	Ciprofloxacin 500 mg orally twice daily
C	Ciprofloxacin 500 mg orally twice daily plus doxycycline 100 mg twice daily
D	Doxycycline 100 mg twice daily for 1 week
E	Gentamicin 1 mg/kg iv
F	Gentamicin 10 mg/kg iv
G	Trimethoprim 200 mg orally once daily
H	Trimethoprim 200 mg orally twice daily

From the list above, select the most appropriate treatment for each of the following clinical scenarios below. The items may be used once, more than once or not at all.

1 A 25-year-old presents to A&E with urethral discharge and dysuria. She uses the combined oral contraceptive pill for contraception. A Gram stain of her urine demonstrates Gram-negative diplococci.

2 A 32-year-old woman is referred to the outpatient clinic with recurrent urinary tract infections, confirmed with positive urine cultures. She has been investigated and no abnormality has been found.

3 An elderly man attends the urology outpatient clinic. He is found to have chronic urinary retention with a bladder palpable to the level of the umbilicus. You arrange his admission for insertion of a urethral catheter.

188 ANTIBIOTICS

1** **C – Ciprofloxacin 500 mg orally twice daily plus doxycycline 100 mg
twice daily**
This is gonococcal urethritis.

2 **G – Trimethoprim 200 mg orally once daily**
For prophylaxis.

3 **E – Gentamicin 1 mg/kg iv**

- See ERN MRCS Book 1, Chapter 11, section 4.

- Treatment for gonorrhoea (Gram-negative diplococci) is ciprofloxacin
  and doxycycline.

- Antibiotics for urinary sepsis are selected on the basis of high
  bioavailability in urine.

- First-line treatment for urinary tract infection is trimethoprim 200 mg
  twice daily, second line is ciprofloxacin 500 mg twice daily, while
  definitive culture and sensitivities are awaited.

- Trimethoprim 200 mg orally once daily is often used for prophylaxis in
  recurrent urinary tract infection.

- Gentamicin cover should be administered whenever instrumentation of
  the urinary tract is performed.

189 THEME: SCROTAL SWELLINGS

A	Congenital communicating hydrocele
B	Direct inguinal hernia
C	Ectopic testis
D	Epididymal cyst
E	Epididymo-orchitis
F	Hydrocele
G	Inguinoscrotal hernia
H	Seminoma
I	Varicocele

From the list above, select the most likely diagnosis for each of the following clinical scenarios below. The items may be used once, more than once or not at all.

1 A 25-year-old man is referred for assessment of a left hemiscrotal swelling. He tells you that it is not present first thing in the morning. In passing, he mentions that he and his wife have been unsuccessfully trying to conceive for 2 years.

2 A 30-year-old man is referred to the outpatient clinic with suspected testicular cancer. On examination, there is a firm, round, mobile 1-cm mass above the testis. The mass transilluminates.

3 A 47-year-old man is referred for a surgical opinion by an A&E SHO. He has a mass confined to the left hemiscrotum, measuring approximately 5 cm in diameter. The testis is **not** palpable separate from it but it does transilluminate.

189 SCROTAL SWELLINGS

1   **H – Varicocele**

2   **D – Epididymal cyst**

3**   **F – Hydrocele**
       Hydrocele of the tunica vaginalis. It is **not** a hernia as you are told that it
       is *confined* to the hemiscrotum.

- See ERN MRCS Book 1, Chapter 11, section 8.4.

- Examination of scrotal swellings is commonly encountered in the clinical
  section (Part IV) of the Intercollegiate MRCS!

- Three points allow a diagnosis to be made in nearly all cases:

    - Is it confined to scrotum (ie can you get above it!)?
    - Can the testis be palpated separate to the lesion?
    - Does it transilluminate?

- Varicoceles are a reversible cause of subfertility. You **must** examine
  patients standing up or the diagnosis will be missed!

- A new varicocele in an older patient may indicate a late renal tumour
  obstructing the renal vein and the gonadal vein.

- Congenital communicating hydroceles are due to a persistent
  communication of the processus vaginalis with the peritoneal cavity.
  Indirect inguinal hernia may subsequently develop into them.

- Hydroceles of the cord or tunica vaginalis may be primary or develop
  secondary to trauma, infection of malignancy.

190 THEME: HEMISCROTAL PAIN

A	Acute epididymo-orchitis
B	Epididymal cyst
C	Mumps orchitis
D	Reactive hydrocele
E	Testicular rupture
F	Torsion of the appendix of Morgagni
G	Torsion of the testis
H	Varicocele

From the list above select the most likely diagnosis for each situation below. The items may be used once, more than once or not at all.

1 A 12-year-old boy attends A&E with acute onset of pain in the right hemiscrotum. He is tachycardic and examination reveals a tender testis with a thickened spermatic cord.

2 A 56-year-old man with a 3-day history of nagging ache in the right hemiscrotum presents to A&E with acute severe pain. He has a history of previous episodes of retention of urine. He is tachycardic and examination reveals a tender testis.

3 A 22-year-old man with a 3-day history of nagging ache in the right hemiscrotum presents to A&E with acute worsening of his pain. He is febrile and tachycardic. Examination reveals a tender testis and cord. He has blood and pus in his urine.

190 HEMISCROTAL PAIN

1   **G – Torsion of the testis**

2   **A – Acute epididymo-orchitis**

3**   **A – Acute epididymo-orchitis**

- See ERN MRCS Book 1, Chapter 11, section 8.4.

- Clearly, testicular torsion is the diagnosis **not** to be missed in such patients!

- This remains a **clinical** diagnosis. If suspected the scrotum **must** be explored!

- If in doubt it is better to explore a normal scrotum than ignore a torted testis.

- Torsion is uncommon in patients of over 35 years of age. Peak age 12–18 years old. It is an acute ischaemic event and may be associated with systemic symptoms.

- Epididymo-orchitis is much commoner in patients over 35 years old, especially those with present/previous urinary sepsis (eg due to prostatic enlargement).

191 THEME: RENAL MASSES

A	Angiomyolipoma
B	Oncocytoma
C	Renal cell carcinoma
D	Renal hydatid cyst
E	Sarcoma
F	Squamous cell carcinoma of the renal pelvis
G	Transitional cell carcinoma of the renal pelvis
H	Wilm's tumour

From the list above, select the single most likely diagnosis for each of the clinical scenarios below. The items may be used once, more than once or not at all.

1 A 35-year-old man, known to have von Hippel–Lindau disease, who has had a previous left nephrectomy for cancer presents with a right-sided loin mass and haematuria.

2 A 3-year-old child presents with an abdominal mass and is found to have microscopic haematuria.

3 A 65-year-old heavy presents with a loin mass. In the past he has had multiple superficial bladder cancers resected and received several courses of BCG. Repeat flexible cystoscopy in the one-stop clinic is normal.

191 RENAL MASSES

1 **C – Renal cell carcinoma**

2 **H – Wilms' tumour**

3** **G – Transitional cell carcinoma of the renal pelvis**
The clue here is the 'field change' effect given previous bladder transitional cell carcinomas.

• See ERN MRCS Book 1, Chapter 11, section 7.1.

• Renal tumours present with renal pain, loin mass or haematuria. Only a proportion of tumours present with all components of this classic triad.

• Urine cytology, ultrasound, CT scanning and/or MRI confirm the diagnosis in most cases.

• von Hippel–Lindau disease is a genetic abnormality that is associated with multiple tumours including renal cell carcinomas (often bilateral!).

• Wilms' tumour (also known as nephroblastoma) is the commonest solid tumour of children.

• Transitional cell carcinoma is thought to occur due to a 'field change' across the entire urothelium. Upper tract tumours are common in patients with multiple recurrences and treatments.

192 THEME: BLADDER CANCER

A   Chemotherapy
B   Intravesical BCG only
C   Intravesical mitomycin C only
D   Neoadjuvant chemotherapy and radical cystectomy
E   Transurethral resection and post-operative intravesical BCG
F   Transurethral resection and post-operative intravesical mitomycin C
G   Transurethral resection only
H   Watchful waiting

From the list above, select the single most appropriate treatment for each of the following clinical scenarios. The items may be used once, more than once or not at all.

1   A patient undergoes a flexible cystoscopy for an incidental finding of microscopic haematuria. There is a solitary red area, which is biopsied. Histopathological examination confirms the presence of transitional cell carcinoma in situ.

2   A 60-year-old man undergoes transurethral resection of several polypoid lesions in the bladder. Histopathological examination confirms the presence of multiple transitional cell carcinomas that are invading through muscle. Staging investigations reveal no evidence of metastasis.

3   A 45-year-old woman is referred for investigation of frank haematuria. At flexible cystoscopy she is found to have several superficial papillary lesions.

192 BLADDER CANCER

1**   **E – Transurethral resection and post-operative intravesical BCG**
Biopsied only at flexible cystoscopy. Thus, needs formal excision.

2   **D – Neoadjuvant chemotherapy and radical cystectomy**

3**   **F – Transurethral resection and post-operative intravesical mitomycin C**

- See ERN MRCS Book 1, Chapter 11, section 7.2.

- Management involves a major distinction between superficial and invasive bladder cancer.

- All new tumours should be treated by resection followed by mitomycin C.

- If they are completely resected then regular subsequent flexible cystoscopy is adequate follow up.

- BCG is used to treat carcinoma in situ following resection of the affected area.

- Invasive cancers may be treated by radical cystectomy or radical radiotherapy.

- Neoadjuvant chemotherapy is with platinum-based agents.

193 THEME: DIAGNOSIS OF URINARY CALCULI

A   Bladder stone
B   Lower calyx renal stone
C   Microlithiasis
D   Prostatic stone
E   Stone at vesicoureteric junction with obstruction
F   Stone at vesicoureteric junction without obstruction
G   Ureteric stone with obstruction
H   Ureteric stone with obstruction and infection
I   Upper ureteric stone without obstruction or infection

From the list above, select the most likely diagnosis for each of the following clinical scenarios. The items may be used once, more than once or not at all.

1   A young woman attends her follow-up appointment in the outpatient clinic. She has a history of mild, intermittent loin pain and haematuria. At her initial consultation, your boss offered her lithotripsy or elective percutaneous removal of her stone. She has opted for lithotripsy.

2   A middle-aged man presents with severe loin pain and rigors. On examination, he is tachycardic and his temperature is 39 °C. He is exquisitely tender in the right loin. His serum creatinine is raised at 210 μmol/l. You admit him for urgent radiological decompression.

3   A young man presents with severe loin pain with nausea and vomiting. The pain is colicky and moves from the loin to settle in the groin. Urine dipstick shows only a trace of blood. IVU shows a delayed nephrogram on the affected side. After 8 hours there is a standing column of contrast all the way along the ureter.

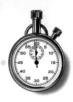

193 DIAGNOSIS OF URINARY CALCULI

1   **B – Lower calyx renal stone**

2   **H – Ureteric stone with obstruction and infection**

3**   **E – Stone at vesicoureteric junction with obstruction**

- See ERN MRCS Book 1, Chapter 11, section 5.
- Stones are formed in the kidney. While they stay there they cause minimal problems (mild loin pain and haematuria). They can be removed electively.
- If they fall into the narrow ureter they cause severe ureteric colic as they pass.
- Calculi tend to obstruct at the narrowest points – ie where the ureter joins the renal pelvis and bladder (the pelviureteric and vesicoureteric junctions, respectively).
- An obstructed kidney has impaired ability to 'take up' and excrete contrast during an IVU, leading to delayed nephrogram and pyelogram/contrast in ureter, respectively. Such abnormalities should thus alert the surgeon that there is (a degree of) obstruction.
- Such features are far more commonly seen on IVU in clinical practice than the much talked about 'standing column'.
- Obstructed, infected systems represent a urological emergency that must be relieved by immediate stent insertion or nephrostomy, as renal function is lost rapidly in this situation.

194 THEME: TREATMENT OF URINARY CALCULI

A	Cystoscopy and JJ stent insertion	E	Percutaneous nephrolithotomy
B	Extracorporeal shock wave	F	Radical nephrectomy
	lithotripsy	G	Simple nephrectomy
C	Flexible ureterorenoscopy	H	Watchful waiting
D	Open pyelolithotomy		

From the list above, select the most appropriate treatment for each of the following clinical scenarios. The items may be used once, more than once or not at all.

1 A 45-year-old man, who speaks no English, is referred by his GP who says that he has a history of kidney stones since childhood. A CT scan reveals a 2-cm stone in the pelviureteric junction on the right. A JJ stent is inserted and a subsequent MAG3 scan demonstrates 95%:5% function left:right kidney.

2 An airline pilot attends A&E where he is found to have a 4-mm stone in his kidney on plain KUB. He is due to fly in 2 days.

3 A 25-year-old man with a 3-mm stone in the mid-ureter has mild obstruction but no signs of sepsis. His pain is reasonably well controlled with simple analgesics.

195 THEME: URINARY TRACT INFECTION

A	*Actinomyces pyogenes*
B	*Chlamydia trachomatis*
C	*Enterococcus faecalis*
D	Methicillin-resistant *Staphylococcus aureus*
E	*Neisseria gonorrhea*
F	*Proteus mirabilis*
G	*Pseudomonas aeruginosa*
H	*Streptococcus pneumoniae*

From the list above, select the most likely causative pathogen for each of the following clinical scenarios. The items may be used once, more than once or not at all.

1 A 27-year-old sexually active man presents with acute epididymo-orchitis. A Gram stain of a urethral smear shows leucocytes but **no** diplococci.

2 A 79-year-old man with a long-history of bladder outflow obstruction and chronic retention of urine secondary to benign prostatic hypertrophy develops epididymo-orchitis.

3 A 54-year-old has bilateral ureteric stents inserted as palliation for advanced cervical cancer. One month later they have become blocked due to 'encrustation'.

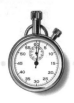

194 TREATMENT OF URINARY CALCULI

1   **G – Simple nephrectomy**

2**   **A – Cystoscopy and JJ stent insertion**

3   **H – Watchful waiting**

- See ERN MRCS Book 1, Chapter 11, section 5.

- Chronic urinary obstruction results in atrophy and loss of function of the kidney.

- A non-functioning kidney should be removed by simple nephrectomy to prevent life threatening sepsis. Radical surgery is reserved for cancer *only*

- A stone of 4–5 mm diameter has a 50% chance of passing spontaneously.

- Obstruction in the absence of sepsis will not cause significant deficit in renal function if it is relieved within 2 weeks.

- A JJ stent will prevent the development of painful ureteric colic and allow the pilot to fly

195 URINARY TRACT INFECTION

1   **B – *Chlamydia trachomatis***

2   **C – *Enterococcus faecalis***

3**   **F – *Proteus mirabilis***

- See ERN MRCS Book 1, Chapter 11, section 5.

- In the young, sexually active patient epididymo-orchitis is usually sexually transmitted. The two commonest pathogens are *Neisseria gonorrhoeae* (Gram-negative diplococcus) and *Chlamydia trachomatis* (not seen on microscopy).

- In the older patient, particularly with chronic urinary retention, the pathogen is usually a bowel commensal.

- Rapid encrustation of urinary prostheses occurs due to the urea-splitting properties of *Proteus mirabilis*, which lowers urinary pH and thus results in precipitation of urinary salts (eg struvite).

196 THEME: CATHETERISATION

A   Condom catheter
B   Indwelling urethral catheter with a flip-flow valve
C   Indwelling urethral catheter with a leg bag
D   Intermittent clean self-catheterisation
E   Latex catheter inserted via suprapubic vesicotomy
F   Mitrofanoff
G   Silicone catheter inserted via suprapubic vesicotomy
H   Tenckhoff catheter

From the list above, select the most appropriate method of urinary drainage for each of the following clinical scenarios. The items may be used once, more than once or not at all.

☐ 1   A quadriplegic patient suffers recurrent problems with his catheter becoming blocked.

☐ 2   A 35-year-old woman develops a neuropathic bladder following attempted surgery for her stress incontinence. She is fully independent and mobile.

☐ 3   An elderly man is acutely confused on account of a urinary tract infection for which he is on correct antibiotic therapy. Unfortunately, although previously fully continent, he has become incontinent. Consequently, the nursing staff ask you to catheterise him. A bladder scan shows that he is adequately emptying his bladder.

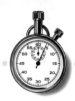

196 CATHETERISATION

1** G – Silicone catheter inserted via suprapubic vesicotomy

2 D – Intermittent clean self-catheterisation

3 A – Condom catheter

- See ERN MRCS Book 1, Chapter 11, sections 6.5 and 6.6.

- The suprapubic route is preferred for patients, particularly female, requiring long-term catheterisation, as it is associated with reduced rates of sepsis further from anus.

- Silicone catheters are more expensive but are designed to resist blockage.

- Intermittent clean self-catheterisation is performed several times per day by the sensible patient with incomplete bladder emptying to facilitate bladder emptying to avoid complications of urinary sepsis and chronic renal failure.

- Colonisation of catheters in the urinary tract occurs rapidly in the presence of infected urine. It is difficult to adequately treat infection in the presence of a prosthesis in the urinary tract, which should thus be removed/avoided if possible.

- Condom catheters are useful in incontinent patients.

INDEX

Note to reader: Entries are indexed by question number, not by page number